Embracing Complexity: Understanding PCOS and ADHD in Relationships

Bradley Hall

Published by Bradley Hall, 2023.

While every precaution has been taken in the preparation of this book, the publisher assumes no responsibility for errors or omissions, or for damages resulting from the use of the information contained herein.

EMBRACING COMPLEXITY: UNDERSTANDING PCOS AND ADHD IN RELATIONSHIPS

First edition. September 25, 2023.

Copyright © 2023 Bradley Hall.

ISBN: 979-8862519228

Written by Bradley Hall.

Table of Contents

This book is dedicated to my wife, Amanda. Without her, this book would not exist.

Introduction

Navigating the intricacies of a romantic relationship takes effort, compassion, and understanding from both partners. When a dual diagnosis of polycystic ovary syndrome (PCOS) and attention deficit hyperactivity disorder (ADHD) enters the dynamic, it can feel like the complexity gets turned up to eleven. As partners strive to support one another through the ups and downs, they are often met with more questions than answers. How exactly do these conditions intersect? What are the most loving ways to communicate about sensitive challenges? Is the frustration and tension a sign that the relationship is doomed?

This book was born from my own journey with my wife, Amanda, who lives with both PCOS and ADHD. When we first met, I was drawn to her quick wit, creative spirit, passion for helping others, and, of course, her beauty. However, as time passed, I realized there were layers beneath the surface I didn't fully grasp—aspects of her health and neurology that profoundly shaped our dynamic. Some days her boundless energy and productivity awed me, while other days her overwhelm and mood crashes left me confused and concerned. Over time, the physical intimacy challenges and emotional volatility strained our relationship and tested my capacity to be an empathetic, understanding partner.

Like many loving partners, I desperately wanted to support Amanda but often felt lost about how to do so effectively. We tended to talk in circles about the same tensions and misunderstandings. My attempts to help—as well-intentioned as they were—sometimes missed the mark or came across critical, leaving her feeling judged. Slowly but surely, I began to withdraw out of exhaustion and frustration. That's when I realized we needed help understanding and embracing the full complexity of the challenges we faced.

Through counseling, support groups, deep listening, and plenty of late-night googling, I gradually discovered resources that helped me better comprehend

Amanda's experiences. As my knowledge grew, so did my ability to meet her in a place of empathy, compassion, and acceptance. My goal in writing "Embracing Complexity" is to share some of the lessons, strategies, and wisdoms I uncovered. My hope is that it will help other partners deepen understanding, enhance communication, navigate challenges with creativity, and build profoundly loving relationships with women who have PCOS and ADHD.

When Amanda was diagnosed with PCOS in her early 20s, all she understood was that it affected her periods and her ability to have children someday. The additional nuances of how PCOS could impact her health holistically or potentially overlap with other conditions were not on her radar. Over a decade later, when ADHD entered the picture, neither of us initially made the connections between her diagnoses. We equated the ADHD primarily to focus challenges and uncontrolled motion rather than recognizing its far-reaching influence.

This book is for any romantic partner—girlfriends, boyfriends, husbands, wives, or spouses—wanting to truly understand how PCOS and ADHD intersect. It's for those yearning to move from feeling baffled, alone, resentful, or burnt out to feeling informed, supported, inspired, and deeply in love. Whether you're new to dealing with these diagnoses or have been navigating them for years, consider this book an accessible guidebook and compassionate friend. It has been cobbled together through notes, research, and several hours of Instagram videos on both topics.

The Path to Diagnosis is Rarely Linear

Amanda's diagnostic journey was complex, as it often is for many women with both PCOS and ADHD. Let's start by understanding some background on these two conditions individually before exploring their intricate interplay.

Unpacking Polycystic Ovary Syndrome (PCOS)

PCOS is a common hormonal and metabolic disorder estimated to impact between 5% to 10% of women of reproductive age. However, many experts believe it is significantly underdiagnosed. PCOS can emerge in adolescence or the early reproductive years, often going undetected for years before diagnosis due to lack of awareness or diverse, fluctuating symptoms.

So what exactly causes PCOS? In basic terms, it stems from a hormonal imbalance, metabolic dysfunction, and genetics. When the ovaries produce excessive male hormones (androgens), it causes irregular ovulation and prevents the ovaries from properly releasing eggs. The follicles in the ovaries then accumulate into cysts. High androgen levels paired with insulin resistance drive many of the symptoms associated with PCOS.

The severity and presentation of PCOS varies widely from person to person. Not all symptoms may be present, which makes detection complex. Classic diagnostic signs include:

- Irregular, infrequent, or absent menstrual periods

- Excess androgens linked to hirsutism (excess body hair growth), alopecia (scalp hair loss), acne, and other skin changes

- Polycystic ovaries visible on an ultrasound

- Metabolic disorders like insulin resistance, obesity, and elevated blood sugar

- Infertility or difficulty getting pregnant

However, PCOS can also cause an array of other symptoms less obviously tied to reproductive health:

- Fatigue

- Anxiety or depression

- Sleep disturbances

- Pelvic pain

- Headaches or migraines

- Slow metabolism and difficulty losing weight

- Darkening skin in creases of the body

- Skin tags

- High cholesterol

The diverse, fluctuating, and multi-system nature of PCOS makes it notoriously challenging to identify. Symptoms often emerge gradually over the course of years. During Amanda's teen years, she experienced severe acne, irregular periods, rapid weight gain, and exhaustion. However, it took until her 20s before a doctor connected all the dots and gave her a PCOS diagnosis. This multi-year diagnostic delay is incredibly common.

In addition to its variable symptoms, there are other reasons why PCOS frequently goes undetected:

- Lack of understanding among patients and doctors

- Symptoms dismissed as separate issues

- Focus only on reproductive symptoms

- Belief it only causes infertility or obesity

- Failure to test androgen levels

- False assumption symptoms will resolve without treatment

- Negative body image avoidance of reproductive health screenings

- Lack of universal consensus on diagnostic criteria

Thankfully, medical understanding and detection rates for PCOS are improving with greater research and awareness. Still, countless women suffer for years before getting answers and appropriate treatment. Many women with PCOS and ADHD separately, have had to go through years, somtimes decades of doctor visits with no idea what causes their symptoms. You can imagine how dificult of a time these people who have both of these diagnoses have had of it.

The additional challenge is that PCOS is not a one-size-fits-all condition. There are four different subtypes reflecting different symptom presentations:

1. Classical PCOS: High androgen levels from the ovaries and small cystic ovaries visible on ultrasound. Most common subtype.
2. Ovulatory PCOS: Normal ovulation and androgen levels but polycystic ovaries on ultrasound.
3. Nonclassical Insulin-Resistant PCOS: No cystic ovaries but symptoms of high insulin and androgen levels like hirsutism.
4. Nonclassical Adrenal PCOS: No cystic ovaries but high male hormones from the adrenal gland.

Given this diversity, PCOS treatment must be tailored to the individual. Lifestyle changes, medication, supplements, diet, and holistic therapies can help manage symptoms. But balancing side effects, costs, and effectiveness takes time and patience. There is no overnight fix.

Introducing Attention Deficit Hyperactivity Disorder (ADHD)

Now let's explore key aspects of ADHD and how this condition intersects with PCOS. ADHD is a neurodevelopmental disorder estimated to impact 8% to 10% of children and around 4% of adults worldwide. However, many experts believe it remains significantly underdiagnosed in girls and women.

The core features involve chronic challenges with inattention, hyperactivity, and impulsivity. ADHD arises from differences in brain structure and chemistry, specifically in regions that govern executive functioning. This includes the prefrontal cortex which oversees planning, prioritizing, organization, regulating emotions, and controlling impulses. Deficits in certain neurotransmitters like dopamine and norepinephrine contribute to many ADHD symptoms as well.

ADHD exists on a spectrum. Not all symptoms may be present, and severity varies. Some key signs and behaviors of inattentive ADHD include:

- Difficulty sustaining focus and easily distracted

- Forgetfulness, missed details, lack of follow through

- Avoidance of tasks requiring sustained mental effort

- Frequently losing or disorganized

- Poor listening skills, mind wandering, zoning out

- Difficulty processing information as quickly or accurately as peers

Signs of hyperactive/impulsive ADHD can include:

- Restlessness, excessive talking, fidgeting, inability to sit still

- Difficulty waiting turns or interrupting others

- Acting without forethought, spur of the moment choices

- Intense impatience, low frustration tolerance

- Excessive and impulsive spending

ADHD often persists from childhood into adulthood. However, symptoms may shift over time. While hyperactivity may decrease, challenges with organization, focus, forgetfulness, and impulse control often continue. Diagnosis typically requires an extensive clinical interview exploring symptoms along with reports from parents, teachers, friends, or partners who interact with the patient in different settings.

Like PCOS, there is no single test to confirm an ADHD diagnosis conclusively. Amanda's journey to getting assessed for ADHD occurred in stages. Iit wasn't until her late 20s that ADHD was explored as a primary diagnosis. Slipping through the diagnostic cracks throughout childhood is very common for girls with ADHD.

Why the Delayed Diagnosis for Women?

There are several reasons why ADHD is underdiagnosed and detected later in life for females:

- Symptoms present differently than in males

- Less hyperactivity and externalized behaviors

- More quiet, inattentive or internalizing traits

- Better ability to mask struggles until adolescent/adult years

- Cultural biases and misunderstanding of female ADHD traits

- Focus on boys with disruptive behaviors in childhood

The less "hyperactive" presentation of ADHD in girls and women often causes their symptoms to be dismissed, undiagnosed, or misdiagnosed well into adulthood. The stereotype persists that ADHD is a disorder of disruptive boys. However, we now know ADHD can manifest very differently across genders.

Additionally, women with undiagnosed ADHD are at elevated risk for developing anxiety, depression, disordered eating, self-esteem issues, and other mental health concerns. These comorbidities result from coping with unrecognized ADHD symptoms for so long without the proper support.

How PCOS and ADHD Intersect

Now that we've reviewed both conditions independently, how exactly can PCOS and ADHD overlap and interact? The connection is still being researched, but several factors are believed to contribute:

Hormonal Influences

- PCOS hormonal imbalances like high testosterone and insulin resistance during puberty may impact brain development.

- Monthly hormone fluctuations through the menstrual cycle can exacerbate ADHD symptoms in women with both conditions.

● ADHD stimulant medications can improve PCOS symptoms like excess hair growth and acne by reducing androgen levels. The reverse is also true: androgen blocking treatments for PCOS can reduce ADHD symptoms.

Genetics

● There are common genetic variants associated with both increased insulin resistance and ADHD risk.

● Up to 20% of women with PCOS have a mother or sister with ADHD.

Obesity

● Insulin resistance promotes weight gain in PCOS and higher BMI is linked to ADHD risk

● Impulsiveness and disorganization from ADHD can disrupt healthy routines needed to manage PCOS-related weight and metabolism challenges.

Mental Health

● The mood instability, anxiety, and depression associated with PCOS may worsen ADHD-related emotional dysregulation.

● Stress exacerbates symptoms of both ADHD and PCOS.

Diagnostic Delay

● ADHD traits of disorganization, lack of follow through, and forgetfulness cause women with PCOS to miss health screenings.

● Missed or absent periods from PCOS mask other symptoms until more severe issues like infertility arise.

- The underdiagnosis of both conditions in women means neither gets properly treated or connected.

In Amanda's case, the signs were there long before her official diagnoses: puberty onset mood swings, volatile emotions, severe adolescent acne, college struggles with focus and procrastination, losing important belongings, traffic accidents from impatience, and longstanding issues with irregular periods, weight gain, and hormone imbalances. However, for years these issues were chalked up to separate causes rather than recognizing the full picture.

Whether related directly through shared genetics or indirectly through behavioral and environmental factors, PCOS and ADHD clearly intersect and influence one another. However, research on this relationship is in early stages, and many physicians are unaware of the overlap. We still have more to learn about how genotypes combine with lifestyle factors in unique ways for each woman. There is no one profile.

For partners, these diagnoses illuminate key areas where targeted support and understanding is needed—from cultivating structured routines to having sensitive conversations about physical intimacy. By arming yourself with knowledge about PCOS, ADHD, and their interplay, you equip yourself to embrace the complexity.

Communication Starts with Listening

"I wish I had listened more closely and understood her better from the beginning."

This sentiment echoes through my early journal entries navigating Amanda's dual diagnoses. In the initial years after her PCOS diagnosis, I would get frustrated by the unpredictable food sensitivities, rollercoaster moods, and peaks and valleys in sexual desire. I didn't have the education or compassion to grasp why she responded so strongly to minor lifestyle tweaks and signals from her body.

Once ADHD entered the picture, I grew annoyed by her chronic lateness, forgetfulness, jumbled piles of paperwork, and constant fidgeting. I took it personally when she got distracted during conversations or missed my cues. My reactions and criticism, while unskillful, came from a place of ignorance. I interpreted differences as flaws instead of opening my mind to understand the root causes.

The Antidote to Ignorance is Insight

But insight cannot take root without first listening to understand, not simply to reply. When we listen half-heartedly, distracted and eager to interject our own thoughts, it blocks us from truly taking in our partner's inner world. We end up glossing over the feelings and perspectives buried beneath the surface words.

Throughout this book, I will refer to treatments and medications that could alieviate some of the symptoms of either PCOS or ADHD. No treatment can be 100% effective at either of these things. I am not giving you medical advice, just showing you that there are options.

Active, non-judgmental listening is like providing rich soil for insight to bloom. Some tips for cultivating deeper listening include:

- Give your partner your full presence and focus. Maintain eye contact. Silence phones. Minimize distractions.

- Reflect back her feelings. "It sounds like you're feeling really anxious and overwhelmed right now. Is that right?"

- Ask thoughtful follow-up questions to understand her experience more deeply. Don't just problem solve.

- Express empathy. Let her know you grasp where she's coming from before offering advice.

- Avoid interrupting or finishing her thoughts. Let her process aloud at her own pace.

- Check your body language and facial expressions. Are you appearing open or closed off?

- Clarify meanings before reacting. "So when you say I'm smothering you, what specifically have I been doing that feels that way?"

When we leap to problem-solving—though well-intended—it can inadvertently minimize emotions. Partners sharing vulnerable feelings want to feel heard and understood first. The solutions can come later.

Of course, listening is a two-way street. We must also share our own inner world and feel genuinely received by our partner. However, when we're in caretaker mode, we often focus exclusively on the other person without voicing our own needs. This builds resentment over time.

Cultivating a Culture of Curiosity

Listening alone isn't enough. We need to approach our partner's diagnoses with openness, curiosity, and a learning mindset. Insight blossoms when we ask thoughtful questions from a place of care.

Amanda once expressed feeling utterly alone and alienated by her dual diagnoses. The more I probed gently, the more I learned of her inner world:

"What's the most isolating part of dealing with both PCOS and ADHD?" I asked.

"Honestly, when I open up to people about either condition on its own, they usually don't get it," Amanda replied. "My friends might know a bit about PCOS as it relates to fertility, but not the other ways it impacts my health and emotions. And any mental health folks I chat with about ADHD get the focus challenges but don't understand the hormone rollercoaster piece."

"That makes total sense" I said, "I can imagine how much more complex it feels having both diagnoses interplaying. Each one has so many layers as it is. That must feel incredibly lonely navigating the intersection without people who fully grasp your experience."

"Exactly," she responded with relief that I empathized. "It's like no one speaks my language or lives on my planet. Each diagnosis has its own challenges, but together they're amplified. I don't feel like I fit into any box or community because of it."

When I leaned into curiosity about her distress rather than pushing solutions, it allowed Amanda to unpack feelings she'd buried for years. I discovered so much about her worldview simply by creating space to listen, reflect, and probe further.

Partners, here are some powerful questions to ask from a stance of care and curiosity:

- How do your PCOS and ADHD symptoms play off one another? What patterns do you notice?

- What's the most misunderstood aspect of your experience that you wish others grasped?

- How do these diagnoses impact how you feel about yourself?

- What support or validation do you most need related to your health conditions that you feel is lacking?

- In what ways do you feel your diagnoses interrupt living life fully or freely?

- When have you felt judged, dismissed, or ashamed due to reactions from others about your PCOS or ADHD?

- What connections between your dual diagnoses might I be missing or not fully appreciating?

When you make space for her authentic feelings and perspectives, it deepens intimacy far beyond problem-solving ever could. She will feel seen, heard, and cared for.

The Path to Compassion is Paved with Patience

"Rushing often hurts more than it helps. Patience is an act of love."

This became my mantra in calming my own frustration.

Understanding PCOS: The Basics and Beyond

When your partner is diagnosed with polycystic ovary syndrome (PCOS), it can feel daunting to grasp everything this complex condition entails. From making sense of ambiguous symptoms to supporting treatment options, PCOS introduces many unknowns. Arm yourself with a strong foundation of knowledge about what contributes to PCOS and how it manifests. Let's delve into the basics of what this syndrome is, why it occurs, and how it impacts health and wellbeing.

We'll also go beyond the surface to explore important lifestyle factors, the diversity of presentations, and advice for empowering your partner. Knowledge breeds compassion, equipping you to embrace PCOS as part of her uniqueness.

Unpacking the Causes: Imbalanced Hormones and Genetics

At its roots, PCOS stems from a hormonal imbalance involving too much of the androgen testosterone. Elevated male hormones prevent regular ovulation, trigger excess hair growth, and contribute to other related issues. Insulin dysregulation also plays a key role. Genetics influence susceptibility, but lifestyle factors determine severity of symptoms.

To understand PCOS, we must first briefly review normal reproductive anatomy and menstrual cycle function. Each month, the hypothalamus and pituitary gland in the brain signal the ovaries to begin maturing a follicle carrying an egg. The follicle grows while releasing estrogen. Mid-cycle, a luteinizing hormone (LH) surge triggers ovulation when the egg ruptures from the follicle.

The empty follicle transforms into the corpus luteum to produce progesterone for thickening the uterine lining. If pregnancy does not occur, estrogen and progesterone levels drop, shedding the uterine lining during your period. Then the cycle repeats.

In PCOS, high testosterone from the ovaries overpowers the signals. Too many follicles start to mature but rarely release eggs. The follicles accumulate into cysts. The lack of ovulation prevents adequate progesterone to balance the estrogen. Irregular shedding of the uterine lining causes infrequent, absent, or prolonged periods.

Insulin further exacerbates this imbalance. Cells become less sensitive to insulin, driving excess production. Excess insulin triggers increased testosterone and hinders ovulation. This vicious cycle underlies the connection between PCOS and metabolic disorders like obesity, diabetes, and infertility.

While the exact causes remain unclear, genetics play a definite role. PCOS appears to run in families, often passed from mother to daughter. Environmental factors like poor diet, stress, and inactivity can worsen genetic susceptibility.

Key Takeaways:

- Excess testosterone is at the root of ovarian cysts and anovulation.

- Insulin dysregulation exacerbates the hormonal imbalance.

- Genetics influence risk but don't guarantee outcome.

- Lifestyle habits significantly shape severity of symptoms.

Understanding the Diverse Symptoms and Health Risks

Now that we've reviewed the hormonal and genetic drivers, let's break down key symptoms that can manifest with PCOS:

Menstrual Irregularities

The most common indicator is irregular, infrequent periods resulting from lack of ovulation. However, cycles can also be very heavy, prolonged, or absent. The uterine lining thickens without bi-monthly shedding.

As a man, it makes sense that I wouldn't know a lot about the entire menstruation process. For other men reading this, you know your wife bleeds every month, or at least is supposed to. With PCOS, this does't always happen, and when it does, it's sometimes unexpected.

Excess Androgens

Elevated testosterone causes hirsutism with coarse hair growth on the face, chest, and belly. Scalp hair loss and acne often occur as well. Darkening skin (acanthosis nigricans) may develop on the neck, under arms, and in skinfolds.

Polycystic Ovaries

Ovarian ultrasound reveals numerous unruptured follicles. The ovaries can enlarge with a classic "necklace string" appearance. However, cystic ovaries alone don't confirm PCOS if other symptoms are missing.

Obesity

Insulin resistance promotes weight gain, predominantly around the belly. However, lean women can have PCOS too. Diet, activity level, and genetics influence body composition.

Fertility Problems

Chronic anovulation prevents regular conception. However, ovulation may occasionally occur without treatment allowing surprise pregnancies. PCOS also heightens gynecological cancer risk.

Metabolic Disorder Risks

Insulin resistance increases chances of impaired glucose tolerance, type 2 diabetes, high blood pressure, and poor cholesterol profiles. These elevate risks for stroke, heart disease, and diabetes complications.

Mental Health Challenges

Hormone fluctuations, body image struggles, pain, and infertility distress can trigger or worsen anxiety and depression for those with PCOS. Studies confirm higher incidence of mood disorders.

As you can see, PCOS is not simply a reproductive disorder. It is a complex endocrine and metabolic condition touching all aspects of health. Symptoms also change over time. Teens may have the worst acne and hair growth while adults struggle more with weight, infertility, and diabetes risk.

This array of possible symptoms combined with gradual onset is why PCOS is so commonly missed or misdiagnosed. Doctors need high clinical suspicion and must take a careful history to connect the dots. Partners can support the diagnostic process by tracking her symptoms long-term and advocating for proper testing.

Testing and Diagnosis: Pinpointing the PCOS Subtype

Since presentations vary, diagnosing PCOS requires a holistic clinical picture, not just one test. Key components include:

Medical History – Symptoms, family history, menstrual patterns, infertility, and lifestyle habits provide clues. Acne, hair growth, obesity, and absent/ irregular periods raise red flags.

Physical Exam – Signs like acanthosis nigricans suggest insulin resistance. Excess facial and body hair point to elevated androgens.

Ultrasound – Imaging reveals ovarian cysts and size. However, alone it doesn't confirm PCOS.

Blood Tests – Labs help identify androgen excess, insulin resistance, inflammation, and rule out related disorders with similar symptoms. Common tests check:

- Testosterone and DHEAS levels

- Fasting glucose and insulin

- Hemoglobin A1C

- Lipid profile

- TSH to assess thyroid function

- Prolactin to check pituitary gland function

- LH and FSH to determine ovulation patterns

Once testing is complete, specific diagnostic criteria include:

- Irregular periods AND evidence of elevated androgens (on exam or labs)

- Polycystic ovaries on ultrasound PLUS signs of androgen excess

However, diagnostic guidelines still vary which contributes to underdiagnosis. The four PCOS subtypes reflect the diversity in presentation:

Classical (Frank) PCOS – High androgens from the ovaries plus ovarian cysts

Ovulatory PCOS – Normal periods but polycystic ovaries with milder androgen excess

Nonclassical Insulin Resistant - Normal ovaries but clear insulin resistance and androgen symptoms

Nonclassical Adrenal – Normal ovaries but excess male hormones from the adrenal glands

Rather than a vague umbrella term of PCOS, identifying the specific drivers and subtype allows for optimal treatment. Work with your partner and her doctor to understand where her symptoms fit.

Lifestyle Approaches: Realistic Expectations

Once diagnosed, many women feel hopeful that lifestyle interventions alone will "cure" their PCOS. They may radically overhaul habits around food, exercise, sleep, and stress management expecting quick fixes. However, PCOS requires a nuanced long-game approach. Patience and compassion are key.

Can nutrition, activity, sleep, and other behaviors positively influence PCOS? Absolutely. A holistic approach enhances any medical treatment. But the severity of someone's symptoms plays a huge role that lifestyle alone cannot necessarily override.

PCOS exists on a spectrum. Someone with mild symptoms may find lifestyle very effective at regulating cycles and androgens. Those with moderate-severe classic PCOS are more likely to need medication along with lifestyle modulation.

Setting realistic expectations prevents self-judgment when lifestyle alone fails to dramatically shift symptoms. Instead, view incremental steps as progress while working closely with her medical team.

Here are some lifestyle measures worth incorporating that may provide benefit:

● Nutrition: A whole foods anti-inflammatory diet rich in vegetables, high fiber carbohydrates, lean proteins, and healthy fats can assist with achieving ideal body composition, balancing blood sugar, improving insulin sensitivity, and reducing inflammation. Avoiding refined carbohydrates, sugary foods/drinks, and saturated fats can help regulate appetite and prevent blood sugar spikes. However, highly restrictive diets tend to backfire long-term for those with PCOS. Work with a dietitian knowledgeable about PCOS.

● Exercise: Regular physical activity, even light movement, can improve insulin sensitivity, aid weight management, reduce inflammation, and boost energy. However, intense exercise tends to over-stress the body and disrupt hormones further. Low to moderate intensity is best – brisk walking, yoga, Pilates, swimming, cycling, light weights, etc.

● Stress Management: Anxiety and chronic stress exacerbate PCOS symptoms by increasing inflammation and insulin resistance. Prioritize adequate sleep, social connection, mindfulness practices like meditation, and loving self-care rituals. Seek counseling if needed for mood issues.

- Targeted Supplements: Specific supplements like inositol, berberine, saw palmetto, and spearmint tea may help mitigate hirsutism, regulate menstrual cycles, aid fertility, support metabolism, and reduce inflammation when used short-term and under medical guidance.

However, supplements are not regulated for safety and quality. Don't expect miracles.

The key is maintaining lifestyle factors within reasonable limits. Drastic measures usually backfire. Small sustainable changes yield the best long-term outcomes.

Medical Management: An Integrative Approach

While lifestyle interventions can be incredibly supportive, most women need some medical treatment to manage PCOS, especially those with moderate-severe classic PCOS. Play an active role with your partner in understanding all options to find the right fit based on symptoms, side effects, costs, and time involved.

Hormonal Birth Control: Oral contraceptive pills (birth control pills) help regulate menstrual cycles and reduce hirsutism and acne by lowering androgens and promoting regular ovulation. However, insulin resistance may worsen with high-dose estrogen containing pills. Lower estrogen options or progesterone-only pills may be preferable for some. Discuss options thoroughly with her doctor.

Fertility Medications: Drugs like clomiphene and letrozole can trigger ovulation in those trying to conceive. Timed intercourse or IUI are often needed. However, fertility drugs increase risk of multiples. IVF with single embryo transfer is sometimes pursued.

Anti-Androgens: Spironolactone blocks androgen receptors reducing excess hair growth, acne, and scalp hair thinning. It has diuretic effects, so electrolytes must be monitored. Topical eflornithine cream inhibits hair follicle enzymes. Laser hair removal can also be effective.

Insulin Sensitizers: Metformin improves insulin resistance, aids weight loss, regulates menstruation, lowers testosterone, and reduces diabetes risk. However, GI side effects are common. Extended release formulations and lower doses help. Pioglitazone and inositol also improve insulin sensitivity.

Mood Stabilizers: Anti-anxiety medications, antidepressants, and anti-seizure drugs may be prescribed short-term for severe PMDD, depression, or anxiety.Improving the hormonal fluctuations can stabilize moods.

Surgery: As a last resort, laparoscopic ovarian drilling can help induce ovulation when other treatments fail. The outpatient procedure uses electrocautery to destroy tissue in the ovaries promoting normal ovulation. However, benefits may be temporary.

Holistic Approaches: Acupuncture, herbal medicine, probiotics, essential oils, light therapy, stress reduction techniques, and targeted supplementation can complement conventional treatments. But always disclose use to your doctor and confirm safety.

While medication and surgery play a role, lifestyle therapy gives the foundation. Work as a team with practitioners utilizing both traditional and holistic modalities to determine optimal individualized management.

Debunking Myths and Empowering Your Partner

Finally, let's explore and debunk some major myths about PCOS. Understanding the facts empowers your partner on her health journey.

Myth: PCOS only causes infertility and obesity.

Fact: PCOS impacts the entire body – hormones, metabolic function, hair growth, skin, mood, sleep, energy, cholesterol, inflammation levels, and much more. It is not defined solely by reproduction and weight.

Myth: PCOS is cured by lifestyle changes or losing weight.

Fact: While lifestyle habits significantly impact PCOS severity, they cannot "cure" it entirely because genetics play a role. However, optimal management integrates nutrition, activity, stress relief, targeted supplementation, and medical therapies.

Myth: Those with PCOS are unhealthy and just need self-control.

Fact: PCOS causes physiological insulin resistance independent of willpower. Those with PCOS need compassion, not judgment about struggles with body composition or motivation. Lifestyle changes can be helpful but never a substitute for medical treatment.

Myth: There's a one-size-fits all treatment for PCOS.

Fact: All manifestations of PCOS are valid – from mild to severe. No singular treatment works for everyone. Combining the right lifestyle plan and medical therapy based on the specific symptoms and drivers is key.

Myth: Only reproductive-aged women get PCOS.

Fact: PCOS can appear any time from menarche into the 40s. Perimenopausal and postmenopausal women can also have lingering metabolic complications. PCOS symptoms change across the lifespan.

Equipped with a thorough understanding of the origins, diagnostic process, diverse symptoms, treatment landscape, and lifestyle impacts, you can truly grasp PCOS' complexities. Avoid myths and assumptions. Instead, approach each unique facet in your partner's PCOS journey with empathy. By embracing her struggles and strengths, you enable growth – as individuals and a team.

The World of ADHD: Breaking Down the Myths

When your partner is diagnosed with ADHD, you may realize how little you know about this often misunderstood disorder. What exactly causes it? How does it manifest differently across genders? Why does it persist into adulthood? What treatments are effective? Let's explore ADHD at a deeper level to grasp your partner's experience.

First, we'll break down the neuroscience and symptoms. Then we'll debunk common myths to empower your partner on her health journey. Knowledge breeds compassion. You may discover ADHD's gifts amidst the struggles, allowing you to celebrate her unique wiring.

Demystifying Causes: Neurotransmitters and Executive Functioning

At its core, ADHD results from atypical brain structure and wiring leading to executive functioning deficits. Certain regions like the prefrontal cortex and networks governing attention, focus, planning, and impulse control don't function optimally. However, there are upsides to the ADHD brain too.

Specifically, low levels of certain neurotransmitters are implicated including:

Dopamine – Regulates motivation, reward-seeking behaviors, motor control, and emotional responses. Low dopamine reduces focus, drive, and learning from consequences.

Norepinephrine – Influences vigilance, alertness, concentration, organization, and regulating emotions. Deficits cause distractibility and disorganization.

Serotonin – Impacts mood, social behaviors, appetite, sleep-wake cycles, and pain perception. Disruption contributes to emotional reactivity and sensory sensitivity.

In those with ADHD, these neurotransmitters don't release optimally in key regions activating the executive networks. As a result, they struggle regulating attention, emotions, impulses, and behaviors essential for goal-directed functioning.

Environmental factors like childhood adversity, substance use, poor sleep, and trauma may further impact neurochemistry and worsen wiring differences in ADHD. However, family history studies confirm genetics play a primary role. Often one or both parents also have an official or unofficial ADHD diagnosis.

Key Brain Differences:

- Smaller prefrontal cortex volume

- Reduced connectivity among executive regions

- Delayed development of inhibition networks

- Atrophy in attention processing areas

- Enlarged reward-seeking circuits

Keep in mind, ADHD differences are not deficits. They represent diverse, creative wiring that can harness unique strengths. Later we'll explore the gifts of the ADHD mind. Right now, let's break down key manifestations.

ADHD Symptoms and Presentations

ADHD behaviors fall into two categories - inattention and hyperactivity/impulsivity. Some display both, called combined presentation. Others only exhibit inattentive traits. Hyperactive/impulsive presentation alone is rare. Around 60% of those with ADHD lean inattentive. Women are more likely to be in this category making their symptoms harder to detect.

Inattentiveness:

- Easily distracted and inability to focus

- Forgetfulness, absentmindedness

- Avoidance of tasks requiring sustained focus

- Failure to follow through, poor organization

- Frequently loses or misplaces items

- Poor listening skills, frequently "tunes out"

- Difficulty completing tasks and remembering instructions

- Difficulty managing time and prioritizing

Hyperactivity:

- Constant motion and restless energy

- Nonstop talking

- Fidgeting, inability to sit still

- Interrupting or blurting out

- Difficulty waiting one's turn

- Excessive and impulsive spending

- Impatience, sensation seeking

- Intrusive behaviors

Symptoms must date back to childhood even if not previously diagnosed. However, hyperactivity tends to decrease with age while inattentiveness persists into adulthood. Other developmental conditions like autism can co-occur or get misdiagnosed as ADHD.

While behaviors manifest across settings, symptoms fluctuate day to day based on circadian rhythms, hormones, stress, activities, and environmental factors. Some days your partner may feel laser focused and calm while other days feel volatile and frenetic. Medication and lifestyle adjustments help stabilize, but some fluctuations will always occur.

Also know that ADHD exists on a spectrum. Your partner likely has traits to milder or greater degrees. There is no absolute threshold where normal behavior crosses into ADHD. Diagnosis depends on the level impairments, struggles, and symptoms negatively impacting her life across domains. Even mild ADHD can disrupt learning, relationships, and performance.

The Gifts of ADHD: Creativity, Intuition, and Passion

While ADHD clearly creates challenges, it also confers unique strengths. Partners should help accentuate these gifts which often lie buried under cultural stigma. Your role is uncovering diamonds amidst the rough edges of disorganization, emotional reactivity, and distraction.

Here are some of the brilliances and superpowers those with ADHD frequently possess:

Big Picture Thinking – They often see the forest while others get lost in the trees. Their minds make novel connections. They generate endless ideas to creatively solve problems.

Innovative Mindset – They question established rules and think outside the box. They brainstorm possibilities rather than following structured formulas. Their minds drift in daydreams where vision is born.

Curiosity and Passion – Their wide interests and enthusiasm infuse activities with joy and meaning. They develop deep expertise from obsessively pursuing passions. Their minds crave novelty.

Sensory Perceptiveness – They notice visual, auditory, and tactile details others miss. This makes them talented artists, designers, musicians, and photographers. Their vivid imaginations transport them.

Relational Intuition – They sense emotions and energy shifts in others with deep empathy. They crave meaningful connection and read subtle social cues.

Improvisation Skills –They thrive on spontaneity. When plans go awry, they improvise creative solutions without rigidity. They live in the moment.

Resilience – They are accustomed to setbacks from an early age. As a result, they develop grit and persistence. They bounce back after failures with commitment to keep trying new approaches.

My wife, Amanda's sensory perceptiveness, curiosity, and passion, led her to the teaching profession, where her improvisation skills helped her teach students the way they needed to be taught, and her big picture thinking allowed her to get a Masters degree in Early Reading and is currently working on a doctoral program in STEM education, where she will be able to teach the next generation of teachers in how to teach science, technology, engineering, and mathematics. Your mileage may vary, but you too have the potential to change the world.

The neurodiversity paradigm views ADHD as an alternative learning style with innate strengths. From enchanted imaginations to lighting fast ideas, the ADHD mind contains gems. When embraced positively, ADHD traits generate growth for both partners.

ADHD Across the Lifespan and Gender Gap

Now that we've explored causes and symptoms, it's important to understand ADHD across the lifespan and gender differences. Many myths persist your partner likely encounters. Let's get the facts straight.

Does ADHD only affect children? Absolutely not! While ADHD may emerge in the early school years, it frequently persists into adolescence and adulthood. In fact, over 50% of children with ADHD continue experiencing symptoms as adults. However, hyperactivity tends to transform into inner restlessness and mental distraction by adulthood. Impulsiveness often improves but remains an issue. Challenges with focus, organization, emotional control, and task completion typically endure and impair life functioning.

Additionally, some adults with ADHD were never diagnosed as kids. Their symptoms were overlooked or misinterpreted, especially in gifted children with good grades. The early struggles attributed to their personality as shy, quirky, or scatterbrained. Often it's not until college when responsibilities mount or adulthood when executive functioning demands peak that impairments prompt diagnosis.

For women specifically, the journey is often even more complex. Why does ADHD get missed or diagnosed years later in girls?

Stereotypes presume boys displaying disruptive, hyperactive behavior have ADHD while quiet, spacey girls are simply daydreamers. However, research confirms the following:

- Girls exhibit less externalizing behavior and more inattentiveness/distraction.

- Their symptoms are mistaken for anxiety, depression, obsessiveness, or quirkiness.

- They use more mental energy to compensate leading to missed diagnosis until exhaustion.

- Their academic struggles get attributed to lack of talent versus neurodifference.

Additionally, girls begin displaying ADHD traits at later ages than boys on average. Puberty's hormonal shift exacerbates distraction, disorganization, restlessness, and emotionality. The decline in academic and social functioning finally prompts assessment in the teen or early adult years.

As a partner, be aware of these gender biases. Track when symptoms arose across her lifespan. Help educate family about manifestations in girls and women that providers historically overlooked. If diagnosed late, support her compassionately as she makes sense of why past struggles were misunderstood. Work together mourning lost time while celebrating present growth.

Treatment Options: Lifestyle, Therapy, Medication, and More

If diagnosed with ADHD as an adult, the next step is exploring treatment options thoughtfully. While no cure exists, identifying optimal management dramatically improves functioning and quality of life. Lifestyle adjustments, counseling, medication, coaching, and alternative therapies all play potential roles.

Psychotherapy – Working with a therapist experienced in adult ADHD equips your partner with coping skills for relationships, work, organization, emotional regulation, and self-esteem. Cognitive behavioral therapy is ideal to alter negative thought patterns and self-talk. Partners can also attend sessions periodically to learn communication and boundary setting tools.

Medications – Stimulant medications like methylphenidates (Ritalin, Concerta) and amphetamines (Adderall, Vyvanse) boost dopamine and norepinephrine in the brain improving focus and attention regulation. However, side effects like appetite suppression, headaches, insomnia, and irritability may occur. Non-stimulants like atomoxetine (Strattera) regulate neurotransmitters while avoiding the highs and crashes. Discuss options and potential risks fully with her prescribing doctor.

Brain Training – Working with a coach on mindfulness practices, cognitive drills, and executive functioning skills can rewire neural pathways. Physical exercise also builds new brain connections. Training the brain's neuroplasticity elicits gradual improvement similar to strengthening muscles.

Alternative Therapies – Healthy nutrition, yoga, acupuncture, massage, biofeedback, neurofeedback, limiting tech time, and improving sleep quality support optimal brain health and self-regulation capacity. While not cured, symptoms can be better managed.

Organization Systems – From wall calendars to digital alerts to color-coding systems, organization tools provide structure and reminders. Visible charts, schedules, and files in easily accessible places allow the ADHD brain to stay on track. Experiment to find which systems work best for your partner's tendencies.

Education/Advocacy – Finally, learning everything possible about ADHD strengthens your partner's self-confidence and ability to educate loved ones. Insight into ADHD as an alternative neurotype bred unique gifts and blindspots. Let go of shame. Advocate for support needs. Share resources to foster understanding. Community delivers comfort.

While medication provides a cornerstone for many with ADHD, optimal outcomes integrate prescription drugs with therapeutic lifestyle techniques and skill building. Patience is key – the right treatment regimen takes months of fine tuning. Schedule frequent check-ins with your partner about what's working, any side effects, and needed adjustments. ADHD management is an evolving process.

Embracing the Positives of Her Neurological Uniqueness

Despite very real struggles, it's important to help your partner embrace the upsides of her ADHD wiring. You can nurture self-confidence and neurodiversity pride. Here are themes to consistently reinforce:

"Your brain just works differently than most." Resist labeling ADHD as abnormal or defective. Highlight that neurodiversity is normal and brings advantages. Use strengths-based language.

"Many of the world's greatest thinkers and innovators also had ADHD minds."

Share examples through history of those who achieved success with ADHD traits. Help put her neurology in a positive context.

"Your passion and creativity are beautiful gifts." Consistently notice and praise the upsides of her mental energy, curiosity, sensorial awareness, and imaginative nature.

"You notice and care about details most people overlook." Appreciate her observational talents, relational intuition, and conscientiousness regarding loved ones' feelings.

"Your spontaneity and flexibility will serve you well."

When plans go awry, praise her ability to improvise solutions and willingness to try new approaches without rigidity.

"Your differences are what make you a creative change agent." Highlight that the world needs her innovation, visionary skills, and rule-breaking thinking.

By reframing deficits as differences, you empower your partner to embrace her ADHD traits with confidence. You help cultivate self-compassion around the struggles by focusing on strengths.

Share resources about successful people with ADHD. Support connecting with ADHD communities. Always speak about her neurology from a lens of possibility not limitation.

Debunking Myths About ADHD: Insights to Share with Loved Ones

Despite expanding knowledge about ADHD, misunderstandings still abound. Let's explore and debunk some major myths plaguing those diagnosed.

Myth: ADHD is the result of bad parenting or a lack of discipline. Children outgrow it by adulthood.

Fact: ADHD stems from neurobiological differences in brain structure and chemistry. While positive parenting helps manage symptoms, it cannot cure or cause ADHD which often persists for life.

Myth: ADHD is over-diagnosed in kids. It's not a real disorder.

Fact: Rigorous assessment is required for diagnosis including psychiatric evaluation, reports from teachers, proof of impairment in learning or activities, and rating scales. Those diagnosed exhibit measurable differences in key brain regions.

Myth: People with ADHD are lazy, unmotivated, or unintelligent.

Fact: When managed properly, those with ADHD can focus for long periods on tasks they find stimulating. ADHD has nothing to do with intellect or desire to achieve. It only impairs regulation of attention and impulses.

Myth: ADHD is the result of poor diet, too much technology/screen time, etc.

Fact: While environmental factors may exacerbate ADHD, they do not cause it. ADHD results from chronic neurotransmitter deficits embedded in brain physiology and genes regulating executive function. It's not a willpower issue.

Myth: ADHD is a childhood disorder. It's rare in girls and adults.

Fact: Over 50% of children with ADHD continue experiencing symptoms as adults. Girls exhibit less hyperactivity but more inattention. Diagnosis in women is delayed due to less disruptive symptoms. Prevalence in adult women is actually similar to men.

Myth: ADHD medication is unsafe long-term or causes drug addiction.

Fact: Stimulant formulations treat ADHD by optimizing neurotransmitter levels in key brain regions. This corrects the deficits driving symptoms. Long term studies confirm meds are safe when taken as prescribed and improve functioning.

By debunking myths and sharing facts, you provide your partner and loved ones with education that dispels judgement. ADHD is a valid neurodevelopmental disorder with evidence-based treatment options. The stigma stems from lack of awareness, not reality. Feel empowered to deliver insights.

Thriving in Love and Partnership

I hope this resource outlining ADHD's origins, science, and solutions provides a helpful starting point for grasping your partner's world. You are embarking together on a journey of nurturing her unique neural wiring – differences and all.

While ADHD poses real challenges, it also confers incredible strengths. By embracing the neurodiversity paradigm, you can help your partner cultivate self-love and confidence. Support her in finding the right professional treatment, community, and lifestyle balance. Exercise patience with the process. And above all, consistently reiterate that her mind is beautifully, wondrously ADHD.

The Intersection: How PCOS Can Intensify ADHD Symptoms

When your partner lives with both polycystic ovary syndrome (PCOS) and attention deficit hyperactivity disorder (ADHD), it's crucial to grasp the intersections. On their own, managing either condition poses challenges. But together, PCOS and ADHD can interact in ways that heighten certain symptoms and impact functioning.

How exactly can PCOS exacerbate ADHD? The connections are multifaceted, involving brain development, hormones, metabolism, genetics, and more. While research on the intersection is still emerging, insights equip you to best support your partner through symptom flares.

Let's explore seven ways PCOS can amplify ADHD symptoms along with tangible tips you can offer to lessen the impact. Growing your knowledge fosters compassion and allows you to be a partner, not just a caretaker.

1. Menstrual Cycle Effects

The hormonal fluctuations of PCOS can intensify ADHD symptoms premenstrually and during periods. Specifically, the changing estrogen and progesterone levels over the course of the menstrual cycle influence dopamine and norepinephrine—key neurotransmitters implicated in ADHD.

As estrogen drops and progesterone rises mid-cycle leading up to a period, dopamine declines. Dopamine is vital for motivation, focus, and impulse control. When dopamine dips too low, common ADHD symptoms like distraction, restlessness, emotional reactivity, and mental fog worsen. Those with PCOS already experience more drastic hormonal ebbs and flows due to irregular ovulation. Combined with ADHD dysregulation, the premenstrual phase becomes the perfect storm.

Research confirms women with ADHD report exacerbation in their symptoms coinciding with the luteal phase of the menstrual cycle when estrogen and dopamine hit their nadir. The cyclic hormone shifts make it harder for those with ADHD to maintain their usual coping skills and function. Your partner likely experiences enhanced mood volatility, inability to focus, disorganization, and sensory sensitivity for 1-2 weeks monthly.

Support Tips:

- Track her cycles and be extra compassionate during the luteal phase (week before period) when symptoms peak. Adjust expectations for her capacity.

- Help devise personalized coping methods – increase exercise, mindfulness/meditation practices, simplify obligations, or utilize productivity tools.

- Discuss medication dosage adjustments with her doctor during symptomatic weeks if ADHD symptoms become unmanageable.

- Ensure good premenstrual nutrition and hydration as blood sugar crashes worsen effects.

1. Insulin Resistance and Obesity

The metabolic dysfunctions of PCOS also exacerbate ADHD impairments. Insulin resistance along with inflammation promote weight gain and obesity in those with PCOS. However, obesity also heightens risk for ADHD through effects on the prefrontal cortex, brain volume, and dopamine levels. The two conditions fuel each other.

Additionally, the impulsivity and disorganization inherent in ADHD sabotage the healthy lifestyle habits needed to manage PCOS weight and metabolic issues. The symptoms of one condition directly worsen the other. It becomes a self-perpetuating cycle.

Research demonstrates that higher body mass index (BMI) is associated with reduced gray matter volume in ADHD brains, particularly in regions like the prefrontal cortex vital for focus, planning, and self-control. Obesity-induced inflammation also impairs cognitive faculties.

Conversely, ADHD-related reward seeking and poor planning drive unbalanced nutrition, skipped workouts, technology overuse, and erratic sleep. Lack of organization and follow through stymie healthy routines to manage insulin resistance. The ADHD-PCOS combo intensifies the metabolic and brain effects of excess weight.

Support Tips:

- Gently encourage regular exercise you can do together such as walks or yoga to impact endorphins, inflammation, and stress.

- Collaborate on ADHD-friendly meal plans and prep strategies focused on whole foods, lean proteins, complex carbs, and fiber.

- Set reminders to take medications, vitamins, or supplements that support metabolic health. Establish cues to refill scripts.

- Help devise organization systems for fitness gear, healthy snacks, cooking tools, or gym bag to ease starting routines. Provide ongoing positive reinforcement.

1. Emotional Dysregulation and Anxiety

The emotional volatility accompanying PCOS can amplify mood symptoms of ADHD. Hormonal swings paired with pain, bloating, sleep loss, and fertility worries provoke irritability, anxiety, sadness, and trouble coping.

Simultaneously, ADHD generates emotional impulsiveness and reactivity from poor inhibition control. Difficulty regulating emotions is a hallmark ADHD trait. When combined with PCOS hormone and metabolic shifts, the result is greater intensity of mood swings, stress, and overwhelm.

Research on this intersection found women with both conditions experience higher rates of anxiety, depression, disordered eating, and emotional outbursts compared to those with only one or none. The dual diagnosis presented the greatest psychiatric symptom severity.

Support Tips:

• Actively listen without judgment when emotions seem irrational. Say "I know this feels especially overwhelming right now. How can I help?"

• Model healthy ways to vent feelings like journaling, calling a friend, or exercising. Suggest calming skills like deep breathing, distraction techniques, or meditation apps.

• If you sense depressive thinking patterns emerging, have an open discussion about seeking therapy and remind her of your unconditional support.

• Help identify potential daily stressors that can be restructured. Protect time for enjoyable hobbies that boost mood.

1. Sleep Disturbances

Both PCOS and ADHD commonly disrupt sleep cycles and quality. When combined, these effects compound leading to greater daytime impairment from exhaustion and mental fog.

Hormonal shifts and cortisol spikes from insulin resistance impair PCOS sleep. Simultaneously, ADHD symptoms like restlessness, hyperactivity, and inability to shut off thoughts interfere with initial sleep and continuity. The processes disruptive to sleep biochemistry differ for each disorder but result in similar dysfunction.

Studies show those with both PCOS and ADHD take longer to fall asleep, experience less restorative REM, and have repeated night wakings. Daytime drowsiness, fatigue, and inattention worsen. Shortened sleep reduces alertness, reaction times, and motivation - exacerbating ADHD impairments.

Support Tips:

- Help implement good sleep hygiene habits – limiting electronics at night, no caffeine after lunch, bedroom media curfews, cool temperature setting.

- Suggest white noise, weighted blankets, blackout curtains, or eye masks to reduce disruptive stimulation.

- Try herbal teas, magnesium supplements, or melatonin with physician guidance and monitoring.

- If sleep remains highly disrupted, ask her provider about temporary sleep medication to reset rhythms.

1. Medication Interactions

Certain prescription drugs used to treat PCOS like metformin can interact with ADHD medications. While rare, it's important to monitor potential side effects.

For example, the stimulant mixed amphetamine salts (Adderall) requires an acidic gut environment to be absorbed optimally. Metformin and other antidiabetic drugs raise gut pH creating a more alkaline environment. As a result, Adderall levels can decline when taken together.

Lower stimulant availability means ADHD symptoms will be less controlled. However, stopping metformin medication will exacerbate PCOS metabolic effects. It's a tricky balance.

Have your partner speak with her prescriber about the best timing strategy for taking these medications to optimize both treatments. For example, dose the Adderall XR early in the morning or midday, and take the metformin with dinner to maximize intestinal absorption of each.

Support Tips:

- Remind your partner to disclose all medications to providers to allow screening for potentially problematic drug interactions.

- Assist in setting phone alerts for medication times if needed to help adhere to dosing schedule.

- Provide reminders to take meds/supplements when preparing to leave home or work.

- Monitor if PCOS or ADHD symptoms seem to worsen and communicate with doctor.

1. Cognitive Function

Research demonstrates women with PCOS perform worse on assessments of processing speed, mental flexibility, executive functioning, and working memory. ADHD alone already impairs these cognitive skills that allow efficient thinking, learning, reasoning, focus, and information retrieval.

When ADHD cognitive deficits interplay with similar dysfunction from PCOS, challenges magnify across all facets of life. The cumulative impact makes it harder to digest instructions, stay attentive in conversations, organize tasks, and complete projects requiring sustained mental energy.

Support Tips:

- Write down multi-step instructions for her and break larger tasks into smaller, distinct chunks to prevent overwhelming.

- Gently guide focus back if you notice her mental attention drifting during important discussions.

- Reduce external stimuli during demanding cognitive work by turning off electronics, closing doors, or suggesting noise-cancelling headphones.

- Offer to track key details during complex conversations and provide recaps rather than relying solely on her recall.

1. Treatment Barriers

The executive functioning dilemmas inherent in ADHD like disorganization, lack of follow through, and forgetfulness interfere with successfully managing PCOS.

For example, those with ADHD often struggle tracking their menstrual cycles, scheduling PCOS-related doctor's appointments, and remembering to take medications consistently. They may procrastinate on ordering prescription refills until it's too late. Impulse spending may divert finances from affording treatments.

Support Tips:

- Set phone alerts and reminders regarding fertility tracking, upcoming appointments, prescription refills, or supplement schedules.

- Offer to schedule medical visits while on the phone if your partner has call avoidance. Join periodically to help track symptoms and ask questions.

- Suggest a wall calendar, vision board, or notes on bathroom mirror/doors as cues for health tasks.

- Take the reins sometimes on ensuring adequate exercise, nutrition, and sleep is occurring when ADHD traits impair consistency.

While PCOS and ADHD certainly each bring their own sets of symptoms and challenges, this list highlights how their intersection can profoundly amplify certain issues. Now equipped with greater insight, you are ready to step in with targeted assistance aligned with your partner's needs. Understanding the "why" behind her struggles fosters true compassion and care.

Hormonal Roller Coasters: Navigating the Emotional Ups and Downs

Coping with the mood swings, anxiety, irritability, and emotional reactivity accompanying your partner's PCOS and ADHD can feel like a rollercoaster. One moment she's laughing and optimistic, the next she's crying or lashing out in anger. When hormones, neurotransmitters, and emotions constantly fluctuate, it makes any relationship turbulent. You ask yourself how much moodiness is justified? How can I help regulate the outbursts and crashes? Why does my reassurance not get through?

This chapter validates how deeply distressing navigating these hormonal and neurological ups and downs can feel. I'll explain the science behind the volatility and offer actionable communication strategies for smoothing the ride. The key is balancing patience and boundary setting with loving encouragement. Master the art of holding space.

Why is Emotional Regulation So Challenging?

To understand your partner's mood swings, you must grasp the bodily systems and brain wiring differences driving them. Let's quickly review:

- PCOS hormone imbalances – especially fluctuating estrogen, progesterone, testosterone, and insulin – destabilize moods across the menstrual cycle.

- ADHD involves innate biochemical differences in brain regions controlling inhibition, focus, and emotional impulses like the prefrontal cortex.

- Nutritional deficiencies, sleep disruptions, stress, and inflammation from both conditions further impair mood-regulating neurotransmitters.

In basic terms, the cyclic hormonal shifts of PCOS impair emotional equilibrium the weeks surrounding ovulation and menstruation. Simultaneously, ADHD wiring makes it harder to control reactions, handle frustration, or avoid emotional overreactions due to deficits in self-inhibition.

Now combine the two – the resulting neurological and endocrine collision generates the highest highs and lowest lows. The diverse mood-altering effects converge to create a perfect storm.

Emotional volatility differs day-to-day for your partner based on many factors:

- Menstrual cycle phase

- Quality of diet, sleep, exercise, and stress management

- ADHD medication timing and dosage

- Current life events or responsibilities

- Interpersonal issues or points of connection with you

As a partner, the most crucial skill you can cultivate is learning her cycles and rhythms – identifying patterns in the chaos. Track her periods, note symptoms, watch for premenstrual tension. Also closely observe lifestyle habits like erratic eating, technology overuse, or missed workouts that tend to precede crashes.

Help her name the feelings beneath the reactivity. "You seem really touchy and on edge the last few days – is sadness or stress also under the surface?" Naming masked emotions defuses intensity.

Slowly but surely you'll anticipate what helps counterbalance the volatility. You'll recognize when patience and space is needed versus firmer boundaries.

Mastering the Art of Holding Space

Regardless what prompts an emotional eruption or breakdown, your most powerful tool is learning to hold space. This means figuratively and literally creating a non-judgmental space for whatever emotions your partner experiences to just be.

It's tempting to reactively problem solve, offer platitudes meant to reassure, or withdraw when things get heated. But resist this urge. Emotional acceptance must come first before solutions.

Holding space is an art requiring mindful, compassionate presence. Silence your inner advisor and critic. Bring full focus to her words and the vulnerable emotions underlying them. Let go of trying to "fix" her feelings. Root yourself in deep listening.

Some phrases that communicate acceptance include:

- "I'm right here with you during this tough moment."

- "It makes total sense this is feeling overwhelming right now."

- "I recognize how distressed/discouraged/angry/unsafe you feel."

- "I'm not going anywhere. Let it all out."

- "You have every right to feel this way. I've got you."

Warmth, understanding, and validation must surround her before logic can get through. Once the intensity passes, that's when you transition to collaborative problem solving:

- "Now that some of the initial rush of emotions has eased, how can I help make things better?"

- "What small step could we take to start shifting this?"

- "You know I'm always in your corner. Let's figure out a solution together."

Holding space sounds simple but requires heroic patience when another's pain triggers your own. Recognize that her sensitivity comes from a place of deficits she cannot simply will away. Your grounded presence balances the volatility.

Managing ADHD Meltdowns with Care

The emotional intensity and reactivity your partner experiences often manifests as full meltdowns with floods of tears, yelling, defensiveness, or shutting down entirely. Meltdowns represent the collision of intense shame, frustration, and feeling completely overwhelmed.

ADHD emotional dysregulation lowers the threshold for what triggers a meltdown reaction. Transitions, interruptions, too much stimulation, disappointment, or perceived failure can all elicit overwhelming sensations.

Meltdowns differ from typical anger outbursts. They often feel physically uncomfortable and disconnect the prefrontal cortex which makes rational processing impossible in the moment. Attempts to logically problem solve will fail.

Your compassion is the life raft during emotional flash floods. Do your best to soften your gaze, keep voice low and calm, offer space if needed, and validate the legitimacy of the feelings. Say "I know this all feels unbearable right now. I've got you. We'll get through this together."

Also pay attention to signs a meltdown may be brewing like emotional sensitivity, sensory overload, forgetting self-care, or burnout signals. Help guide your partner through preventive skills like:

- Taking a break in a quiet space

- Going for a walk or doing jumping jacks

- Calling a friend

- Diffusing essential oils

- Yoga stretches or meditation

- Cuddling a pet

- Listening to music

Over time you'll learn cues for when to gently encourage these coping tools. It may prevent full-blown meltdowns.

Healthy Conflict vs Toxic Fighting

Along with emotional reactivity, the mood effects of PCOS and ADHD also negatively impact conflict resolution. Minor disagreements or misunderstandings easily escalate into toxic fighting. Volatility undermines trust.

However, some conflict is healthy and inevitable. The key is communicating through issues productively. Reframe arguments as catalysts for intimacy, not reasons to withdraw. Here are tips to transform fights from toxic to productive:

Don't entirely avoid conflict – Suppressing tensions breeds resentment. But approach sensitive conversations when you're both calm and alert. Don't pick fights when sleep deprived, hungry, or hormonally off-balance.

Discuss one topic at a time – Don't spiral into airing every grievance. Isolate individual issues needing compromise. If emotions heighten, take a 30 minute breather before resuming.

Listen thoroughly before responding – Really absorb her words and reflect them back to ensure you understand her perspective before reacting defensively.

Express yourself without blaming – Use "I" statements about your needs rather than "you" statements with accusations. Take ownership of your feelings.

Validate each other's experience – Don't minimize or dismiss your partner's feelings. But also don't accept unfair blame. Seek collaborative solutions.

Avoid mean statements you'll regret – Don't shame, ridicule, or intentionally] hurt your partner. Focus on resolving the conflict, not winning an argument.

Negotiate compromises – Be willing to meet halfway rather than defending extreme positions. Compromise makes you partners through problems.

Learn when to take a break – If anger escalates unproductively, call a time out. Separate until calm. Temporarily withdrawing is okay if you commit to later reconciliation.

Forgive easily – Don't hold grudges or keep score after clashes. Drop the need to be "right." Assume positive intent from your partner.

While bumps are normal, ultimately both people must feel safe, respected, heard, and loved after conflicts for the relationship to thrive. Reflect on your communication patterns after disagreements. Do discussions repair connection or breed disconnection? All couples must continually refine their comfort with emotional expression.

When Mental Health Suffers: Getting Help

Despite your best support efforts as a partner, the dual forces of PCOS and ADHD may profoundly impact your partner's mental health and self-esteem. Mood disorders like depression or anxiety often accompany these conditions. Partners can only do so much mitigating the effects. Professional help is frequently needed.

Look for persistent signs like:

- Loss of pleasure/interest in most activities

- Appetite and sleep changes

- Social withdrawal and isolation

- Fatigue, agitation, or mental sluggishness

- Feelings of worthlessness, guilt, or hopelessness

- Difficulty concentrating or making choices

- Thoughts of death, self-harm, or suicide

Don't hesitate to gently raise concerns coming from a place of care. Make it conversation, not confrontation or criticism.

"I've noticed you seem really down and disengaged lately. I think life has just been so stressful that it's impacting your mood. Maybe talking to a professional counselor for a little bit would help?"

"I love you and just want to make sure you have the support you need. I think a therapist could have some useful ideas for managing the anxiety. I could help you find someone."

Also share your observations with her physician. With both permission and privacy, anytime you suspect real mental health impairment, notify her prescriber. Her provider can screen for depression or anxiety and suggest next steps.

While stigma remains, mental health therapy helps reframe thoughts, build coping skills, adjust lifestyle habits, and often provide medication if indicated. You may attend the occasional session to deepen understanding.

Most importantly, continue reassuring your partner that you take her mental health struggles seriously. Her symptoms are real, not imagined or exaggerated. Help is available, and you are fully supportive of her seeking treatment. Share stories of others who have been helped by therapy. This encourages getting the assistance needed to enjoy life again.

Navigating the Darkness with Empathy

When in the depths of depression, moodiness, or rage, your partner likely feels compelled to frequently vocalize just how terrible she feels. But constant negative emotions drain your compassion reserves overtime. Her darkness threatens to pull you under.

Setting boundaries around emotional processing is wise. Without withdrawing support, you can still request limits.

"I want to be here for you, but we've been discussing the same worrisome thoughts for hours. Let's take a 30 minute break to clear our heads and come back with fresh eyes."

"I know you're hurting. Can we set aside time twice a week to really talk it through where you can vent fully? But go a bit easier on me the other days?"

As an empathetic partner, you must care for your own mental health too. Protect your light. Seek personal counseling if your partner's struggles drag you down. Maintain friends and hobbies that rejuvenate you. You can support her best with your own oxygen mask securely fastened first.

Helping Her Embrace the Magic and the Madness

Finally, an essential role you play is helping your partner embrace the full spectrum of her being – the bliss and the bitterness. Her diagnoses explain the sadness, but inside also lies profound beauty, talents, and light. Remind her often.

When hormonal dysregulation and ADHD emotionality threaten her self-worth,your words can powerfully reframe the madness as necessary counterpart to the magic within her.

Some perspectives to share:

"I know the intensity feels too much sometimes, but that same sensitivity lets you feel things so deeply."

"The hormone shifts are outside your control, but how gracefully you manage them shows your strength."

"The lows make the highs feel that much more vibrant. You appreciate joy because you've known despair."

"Your unique wiring allows you to create art, grasp concepts, and feel empathy unlike anyone else."

"The way your brain works differently is exactly what makes you special, interesting, and compassionate."

With consistent validation about her wholeness, she can learn self-acceptance even on the hard days. Help her trust that no matter how gloomy life feels, brighter moments always return. The light never fully leaves. There is beauty inside even her most beautiful mess.

Focus, Energy, and Distraction: The ADHD Dimension in Relationships

The symptoms of attention deficit hyperactivity disorder (ADHD) introduce unique dynamics into romantic relationships. Core ADHD impairments like distractibility, restlessness, disorganization, and impulsiveness often impact connectedness, communication, and rapport.

As a supportive partner, you can thoughtfully navigate these challenges through education, lifestyle changes, and honing relationship skills. With compassion and teamwork, you'll discover new ways to connect amidst the disconnections.

Why Does ADHD Impair Focus?

To grasp why your partner struggles tuning in, you must understand ADHD's neurological underpinnings. Certain brain regions like the prefrontal cortex governing executive functions are structurally different. Deficits in dopamine, norepinephrine, and serotonin impair concentration abilities.

Specifically, those with ADHD exhibit reduced electrical activity in brain networks linked to external focus and attention. They require extra stimulation to boost engagement. Subconsciously, their minds seek novelty, making sustained interest difficult.

Does this absolve rude zoning out or forgetting important discussions? Of course not. But it reveals why you can't take distraction personally. Your partner isn't purposefully ignoring you or needs to "try harder". Her brain is wired to drift. Have realistic expectations knowing focus fluctuates.

You can help counteract distracting forces using strategies like:

Remove extra stimuli – Turn off TVs and phones. Avoid crowded noisy spots. Declutter surroundings. Silence removes competing stimuli pulling her attention.

Make eye contact – Gently guide her gaze back to you if it wanders. Eye contact anchors focus. But avoid staring contests which can feel confrontational.

Have fidget/tactile toys – Allow doodling, knitting, stress balls, or other tactile objects during discussions to channel excess energy.

Take breaks – Long conversations may require breaks to recharge concentration. Take a quick walk then resume.

Summarize key points – At the end, recap important details, requests, or next steps requiring her focus. Memory challenges necessitate concise summaries.

You must also have patience when your partner seems perpetually "in her own little world". Remember, her mind works overtime. Allow mental meandering without judgement. With compassion and communication, you can regularly reconnect.

Why the Constant Motion and Restlessness?

The turbo-charged engines of an ADHD mind crave perpetual motion and novelty. Seemingly endless restless energy stems from innate neurochemical differences. But practical outlets for motion prevent disruptive impulses.

Specifically, low dopamine and norepinephrine reduce motivation thresholds, making it harder to endure boredom. The brain seeks activation. Ensure regular energetic activities release pent-up drive in healthy ways.

Explore options like:

- Brisk walking, jogging, swimming

- Motor coordination activities – tennis, bowling, skating, martial arts

- Dancing, yoga, pilates

- Hiking, rock climbing, kayaking

- Calisthenics or light weights

Any heart-pumping exercise improves focus, mood, stress levels, and sleep quality as well. Assist your partner in establishing a regimen bundling the physical and mental perks. But avoid overexertion leading to adrenal burnout. Find a sustainable rhythm.

You can expect some level of constant fidgeting, foot tapping, and doodling due to restless wiring. Gently help redirect when it becomes disruptive through touch, embracing, or reminders. With creativity, even restless traits strengthen bonds.

Why So Easily Distracted During Conversations?

Distracted listening often stems from ADHD minds overworking to compensate for attention deficits. Multitasking places excess load on working memory needed to absorb and process information. Listening with full presence requires reining in the urge to redirect focus.

Easy distraction leaves you feeling unheard. Your partner forgets requests, misses emotional cues, or needs constant repeating. Patience with frequent redirection helps. Also beware interpreting distraction as disinterest.

Strategies like the following improve communication:

- Remove clutter/electronics from the conversation space

- Maintain light eye contact, but not to an uncomfortable degree

- Provide fidget toys to occupy hands/feet

- Gently reorient attention if you notice it drift

- Cover one topic at a time

- Offer to jot down notes or text key things needing memory retention

- Share vulnerable feelings at times when she seems most relaxed and focused

You may need to let go of expecting perfect active listening. Allow stress-free mental wandering during lighter discussions. Judge less when having to repeat yourself frequently. Framing ADHD traits through a lens of understanding prevents building resentment.

Navigating Hyperfocus: The Superpower and Kryptonite

While ADHD clearly causes attention challenges, many with ADHD also hyperfocus at times. They fixate on specific topics, projects, or hobbies with long-lasting zeal. Hyperfocus represents both an incredible gift and relationship double-edged sword.

When channeled productively, hyperfocus enables partners with ADHD to tap into genius states of flow, creativity, and obsession over their passions. However, it also leads to:

- Forgetting other obligations or feeling unable to shift tasks

- Becoming so absorbed they block out the outside world

- Irritability when broken from trance-like concentration

- Neglecting basic needs like eating, sleeping, or socializing

The intensity of hyperfocus helps partners with ADHD excel professionally and cognitively. However, understand it may also periodically disrupt connecting. Avoid nagging to simply "pay attention." Instead, politely offer activities aligning with her passions as pleasing distractions. With care, you can gain skill utilizing hyperfocus as a relationship superpower when it activates.

Managing Impulsive Behaviors

Impulsiveness involves acting spontaneously without adequately considering consequences. It manifests in spending, eating, interpersonal interactions, and risk-taking. Impulsivity arises in ADHD from poor communication between regions that govern motivation and those that inhibit behavior.

To support your partner, establish mutually agreed upon systems creating helpful pauses before impulses run free. For example:

Finances – Institute waiting periods for large purchases, automated savings/bill pay, required discussion of big expenses.

Projects – List pros/cons before launching new endeavors. Set reminders to complete existing tasks before moving onto shinier ones.

Diet – Meal prep together and keep healthy snacks on hand to avoid impulse eating.

Socializing – Before responding to irritating messages/comments, practice taking a few breaths to react calmly.

Risky behaviors – Discuss reasonable limits on things like alcohol, drugs, gambling, speeding etc. based on past issues. Sensitively share concerns.

Sex – When initiation seems impulsive versus mutual, redirect to activities fostering intimacy and bonding first.

Approach limiting impulsiveness as a team effort, not policing. Because ADHD involves developmental delay in the brain's self-control regions, your support scaffolding those areas reduces shame. Setbacks will occur but move forward with patience.

Why the Excessive Energy and Talkativeness?

The innate vigor and enthusiasm of an ADHD mind often manifests in effusive conversation styles. Partners may feel constantly interrupted, talked over, or bombarded with a stream of thoughts without room for input. But there are communication approaches to balance this energy.

Rapid speech and excessive verbiage stem from under-developed mental filters combined with racing thoughts. The mind produces more ideas than the mouth can contain. Without judgment, find polite ways to help your partner pause and allow dialogue exchange:

- "You're sharing so many interesting thoughts! My brain can only hold so much at once. Let's chat back and forth so I can process too."

- "I want us both to have a chance to share. Can we take turns and not interrupt each other?"

- "I totally understand your excitement but need a minute to catch up."

- Gently interject with points while she pauses to breathe in her monologue.

- Suggest scribbling down thoughts racing too fast to voice. Some may be worth revisiting.

- If too overstimulated by the pace, request taking a break to digest the conversation before continuing.

With playfulness and empathy, you can create opportunities for balanced exchange. Your partner's enthusiasm enriches discussions when contained constructively. Offer guidance, not criticism.

Why So Much Mental Clutter and Disorganization?

Partners with ADHD often feel plagued by physical clutter and mental disorganization. Their homes, cars, and minds brim with piles of unfinished business. But certain strategies help instill order amidst the chaos.

At the root, ADHD executive functioning deficits make tasks like sorting, scheduling, categorizing and creating systems very difficult. Their busy brains also struggle retaining mental lists. External structure compensates for internal disorder.

Rather than criticizing messiness, design functional systems together:

- Use wall calendars, white boards, and reminders to map upcoming tasks and appointments.

- Sort mail and paperwork into digital or physical file folders for bills, receipts, and records.

- Institute a launch pad near the door to collect items needing removal daily like keys, bags, dog leashes.

- Create specific homes for routinely misplaced items like phones, wallets, and glasses.

- Set phone alerts for daily routines, medication times, or bill payments.

- Schedule 10-15 minutes nightly or weekly for tidying and organizing. Many hands make light work.

While your partner's distractibility and disorganization causes frustration, remember it is not intentional forgetfulness or laziness. ADHD requires different living strategies. Thoughtfully design external structure together to support areas where internal regulation is challenging. Patience is key.

Embracing Spontaneity, Intuition and Excitement

The downsides of your partner's ADHD traits often grab your attention. But remember, locked inside that wandering mind are also incredible strengths. Reframing ADHD forms deeper empathy.

For example, the spontaneity and novelty seeking you may view as distractibility also allows out-of-the-box thinking. Your partner likely:

- Notices creative connections and interdisciplinary insights you miss

- Generates innovative solutions and pushes beyond limits

- Finds joy and humor in unexpected moments

- Actively listens with her full, open-minded presence

- Makes you feel uniquely seen and understood

- Infuses life with passion, humor, and color

Every quality has two sides. The sensitivity you perceive as volatility also makes your partner extra caring. The hyperactivity you view as restlessness provides endless enthusiasm.

Work together to channel ADHD traits into assets. Align focus with purposeful goals. Direct manic energy into athletic activities. Have her write down racing thoughts to harvest innovation.

By truly knowing your partner's ADHD wiring, you learn to communicate in ways that minimize conflicts. You talk less, listen more. You parent or shame less, understand more. You demand less, encourage more. You criticize less, compliment more.

With knowledge comes power – the power to foster a relationship that celebrates rather than constrains your partner's unique spirit. You have so much to teach one another if you let ADHD untie your hands, not bind you. Seek support when needed, but avoid letting others dictate limits.

At the end of the day, embrace that ADHD is not a "condition", but simply a different neurologic operating system. Respect it fully. Thrive together by planning accordingly. Help your partner feel empowered, not inhibited by her mind. This is your shared journey now.

The Role of Diet: Nutrition's Impact on PCOS and ADHD

The food we eat provides the raw materials that fuel our body and brain. Optimal nutrition stabilizes blood sugar, sharpens focus, lifts mood, eases inflammation, and confers energy. Strategic dietary choices can profoundly improve symptoms for those managing health conditions like PCOS and ADHD.

However, there is no universally ideal diet for these disorders. Each individual requires a tailored nutrition plan based on symptoms, metabolism, preferences, and sensitivities. As a partner, avoid dogmatic food rules. Instead help devise a personalized diet that enhances how your loved one feels physically and mentally while still enjoying meals. Let's explore smart strategies for harnessing the power of nutrition.

General Dietary Strategies for Balancing PCOS

Since insulin dysregulation drives many PCOS symptoms, balancing blood sugar through diet ranks among the top lifestyle measures. However, radical restriction tends to backfire. A balanced approach prevents rebounds. Here are some overarching guidelines:

Emphasize whole, unprocessed foods – Focus on quality carbohydrates from fruits, vegetables, legumes, whole grains and healthy fats from nuts, seeds, avocado, olive oil. Limit refined carbs, sugars, saturated fats which spike blood sugar.

Moderate Carb Intake – Avoid drastic low carb or keto diets. About 45-65% carbs from fibrous whole food sources helps sustain energy while stabilizing blood sugar. Match carbohydrate portions to activity levels.

Increase Fiber – 30-40g fiber daily from vegetables, fruits, whole grains, nuts/ seeds optimizes digestion and insulin response.

Prioritize Lean Protein – Moderate protein portions (0.8-1g/kg body weight) curb hunger while preserving muscle tissue during weight loss. Include plant-based and high quality animal proteins.

Eat Regularly – Grazing frequently on small meals/snacks prevents energy crashes and binge tendencies. Time nutrients to fuel activities and workouts.

Stay Hydrated - Drink ample water between meals. Dehydration exacerbates PCOS symptoms like fatigue, mood swings, and mental fog. Herbal tea offers benefits too.

Mind Portions – Even with wholesome choices, excess caloric intake promotes weight gain. Be aware of overeating at meals or needless snacking from habit not hunger.

Limit Alcohol – Heavy regular alcohol consumption strains the liver, stresses hormones, and makes blood sugar control challenging.

Customize Caffeine – Coffee offers antioxidants but excess caffeine stresses the adrenals worsening fatigue and anxiety. Limit to 1-2 moderate cups earlier in the day.

Reduce Salt – Excess sodium exacerbates bloating, fluid retention, and blood pressure often high in PCOS. Cook with fresh herbs/spices instead for flavor.

Address Individual Triggers – Track if any particular foods consistently worsen personal symptoms like acne, hair growth, bloating, or cramps and limit those. Common triggers include dairy, gluten, soy.

Allow Occasional Indulgences – Deprivation backfires. Satisfy occasional cravings for favorite treats in moderation. Just don't let splurges become daily habits.

Make Changes Gradually – Radical restrictions overwhelm. Transition diet in progressive phases, not overnight. Focus on adding in nourishing foods rather than just eliminating "bad" foods.

Patience and flexibility prevents reactive yo-yo dieting. Regard nutrition as one component of a holistic PCOS management plan.

ADHD Dietary Strategies: Matching Meals to Mental Needs

While no specific diet definitively controls ADHD, certain dietary factors seem to worsen symptoms for some individuals. Strategic nutrition tailored to your partner's needs enhances focus, learning, memory, and impulse control.

Stabilize Blood Sugar – Like diabetes management, steady glycemic control prevents energy/mood highs and crashes worsening distraction, anxiety, and hyperactivity. Eat small frequent meals with a balance of smart carbs, fiber, protein and fat. Stay hydrated.

Consider Elimination Trials – If ADHD symptoms seem worse after certain foods, track potential triggers like gluten, dairy, or dyes/preservatives. Try eliminating suspects for 2-3 weeks to assess changes. Reintroduce later to confirm effects. Consult an RD.

Supplement Smartly – General vitamin/mineral deficiencies can exacerbate ADHD impairments. Have your partner's physician test levels of iron, zinc, vitamin D, B vitamins, omega-3s, magnesium and supplement if low based on lab work. Don't megadose recklessly.

Limit Refined Carbs/Sugars – Heavily processed grains, breads, snacks quickly spike and crash blood sugar and energy. Focus on whole grains, fruits/veggies, nuts, seeds, legumes for fiber-rich carbohydrate sources.

Minimize Artificial Ingredients – Food dyes, flavors, sweeteners, and preservatives appear to negatively impact some people with ADHD. Stick to whole foods without additives when possible.

Ensure Adequate Protein – Starting the day with a breakfast containing protein stabilizes energy and cognition better than pure carbs. Incorporate eggs, Greek yogurt, nut butter, beans, or fish.

Always Eat Breakfast – Skipping breakfast leads to distractibility, restlessness, and mental fog. Refuel first thing to replenish glucose after fasting through the night.

Stay Hydrated – Dehydration exacerbates ADHD struggles with focus, memory, and fatigue. Sip water consistently, especially first thing in the morning and during mentally demanding tasks.

Limit Caffeine – While modest caffeine boosts focus initially, excess strains the adrenals and worsens sleep troubles common with ADHD. Avoid after lunchtime.

Minimize Alcohol – Alcohol's sedative effects worsen ADHD inattention, spatial skills, and memory. It also reduces sleep quality and medication effectiveness. Limit intake.

Track Symptom Links – Notice if certain foods consistently help or hinder your partner's ADHD symptoms and adjust intake accordingly. Individual sensitivities vary.

An elimination diet temporarily removing potentially problematic foods followed by slow reintroduction identifies personal ADHD diet triggers. However, consult a registered dietician to ensure adequate nutrition if eliminating entire food groups.

Addressing Insulin Resistance and Weight Management

Since PCOS involves insulin dysregulation and weight gain, slow steady fat loss through caloric balance improves symptoms. However, radical restriction backfires long-term. Have realistic expectations about the pace of loss to prevent self-judgment.

Set Reasonable Goals – Aim for gradual loss averaging 1-2 pounds weekly through modest calorie reduction combined with more activity. Fast drastic loss is rarely sustainable.

Focus on Measurements, Not Just Scale – Muscle gain during exercise can offset fat loss on the scale initially. Assess progress via body measurements, clothing fit ease, energy levels, cycle regulation etc.

Calculate Needs – Use calorie calculators to determine maintenance level based on age, weight, activity and gently reduce from there. Deficits over 500 calories daily usually rebound.

Track Intake – Logging meals provides awareness of calories, nutrients, and habits. Note hunger levels across the day. Many smartphone apps help with tracking.

Beware Extreme Low Calorie Diets – Very low calorie plans strain hormones, sap energy, and deplete muscle long-term. Slower loss through modest reduction feels more sustainable.

Emphasize Nutrient Density – Focus diet on nourishing whole foods packed with antioxidants, fiber, protein, and healthy fats to prevent feeling deprived. Frozen, canned, and bagged options work too.

Combine with Movement – Any activity level safely boosts caloric needs making weight management easier. Find enjoyable consistent workouts. Even light exercise helps insulin sensitivity.

Practice Mindfulness – Tune into body signals for genuine hunger versus just boredom or stress eating. Does the body need fuel or are you eating from habit?

Forgive Lapses – Perfection is impossible. Slip ups are learning opportunities about triggers. Get back on track at the next meal, not next week. Progress trumps perfection.

Surround with Support – Tackle lifestyle changes together as a team. Help meal prep. Remind about goals. Provide positive praise. But avoid policing.

Be Patient – If progress stalls, wait it out 1-2 weeks before adjusting calories further. Our bodies judiciously adapt to change. Trust the process.

Sustainable weight loss for PCOS requires partnership - an intimate team effort not an individual burden. Take care of emotional needs too by staying connected to community, self-care practices, and counseling if helpful. Diet alone cannot cure PCOS but nourishing the body empowers the whole person.

Meal Planning Strategies for Two

Planning ahead takes the stress out of nourishing meal prep. No more scrambling last minute or grabbing takeout. Get creative with food and have fun trying new flavors recipes together. Some tips:

Do Weekly Meal Planning Sessions – Browse cookbooks/blogs and grocery flyers together for inspiration. Draft meals for the week ahead including 2-3 simple weekday dishes and 2 more elaborate weekend ones.

Make Detailed Shopping Lists – Compile needed ingredients for planned recipes as well as healthy staples and snacks. Shop with list in hand to prevent impulse buys.

Assign Roles – Share the tasks from menu planning to grocery shopping to actual cooking. Play to your strengths. Teach each other new techniques.

Prep Ingredients In Advance – Take 15 minutes after shopping to wash, chop, portion veggies and pre-cook grains. This allows tossing together meals easily.

Cook Extra - Make double batches when possible then freeze individual parts. Reheat for quick meals later. Leftovers become lunches.

Keep It Simple – Focus on meals with 5 ingredients or less, single pot/pan/ baking sheet for easy cleanup, and < 30 minutes hands-on time. You'll cook more with less hassle.

Focus on Produce – Shop seasonally and let veggies/fruit inspire meals. Fill half your plate with plants for volume and nutrients. Keep fresh washed and cut handy for snacks.

Satisfy Cravings - Don't ban all treats. Indulge occasionally in smaller portions. Or find healthier swaps like banana ice cream or cauliflower pizza crust. Just balance sweets with nutrition.

Make Portions Automatic – Use portion control dinnerware or food storage containers to assemble meals with perfect macros/calories for your goals. No counting or measuring needed.

Batch Freeze Extras – Frozen individual meal/snack portions provide grab and go options for busy days. Ideas include soup, chili, muffins, healthy homemade frozen meals.

When you systemize nutrition instead of winging it meal to meal, you reduce decision fatigue and conflicting needs. With collaboration, you can craft a diet optimal for both your health conditions and relationship.

Navigating Food Sensitivities

Many partners with PCOS and ADHD report worsening of symptoms when eating certain trigger foods like dairy, gluten, or soy despite not having a diagnosed allergy or intolerance.

Overlapping digestive issues like irritable bowel syndrome (IBS) or small intestinal bacterial overgrowth (SIBO) aggravate sensitivity. Trialing an elimination diet helps identify personal problem foods.

Exclude Suspect Foods – Based on your partner's observations, cut out potential triggers completely for 3-4 weeks. Common culprits include dairy, gluten, grains, legumes, nightshades, artificial sweeteners.

Read Labels – Check processed foods for hidden sources like whey, malt flavors, vegetable proteins etc. Stick to basic whole foods during elimination.

Track Symptoms – Note changes like digestion, bowel movements, brain fog, energy, pain, focus etc. after eliminating triggers.

Add Triggers Back Slowly – After the exclusion period, add one food group back every 3 days observing effects. Take detailed notes.

Range of Reactions – Look for symptoms both immediately after eating triggers and delayed like worsening eczema, anxiety, insomnia, concentration issues a day later indicating food reactions.

Rotate Problematic Foods – If only able to tolerate triggers infrequently, avoid consecutive days eating them. Follow pizza with a salad day.

Supplement Strategically – Talk to your healthcare provider about digestive enzymes, probiotics, L-glutamine, quercetin or videos to support gut lining health and reduce systemic immune reactions to food compounds.

Work with a Dietitian – Get guidance tailoring your diet to ensure nutritional adequacy if excluding multiple food groups long-term. Prioritize diet diversity.

Pay close attention to how your partner feels before and after meals to pinpoint triggers. Keep an open mind - sensitivities develop at any time even to previously safe foods. Patience, self-compassion, and teamwork help navigate the tricky but important discovery process.

The Gut-Brain Connection

Emerging research reveals important links between gut health and brain function. The enteric nervous system lining the digestive tract actually contains as many neurotransmitters as the brain. The gut microbiome - trillions of bacteria residing there – also constantly impact cognition and mental health. Optimizing the gut-brain axis through diet and supplements sharpens focus, improves mood, and reduces inflammation.

Eat More Fermented Foods – Sauerkraut, kimchi, kefir, yogurt, tempeh, miso contain beneficial probiotics that populate gut flora. Or take high quality probiotic capsules.

Increase Prebiotic Fiber – Asparagus, garlic, onion, tomatoes, bananas, oats feed healthy gut bacteria. Aim for 5-10 grams of fiber per meal.

Drink Bone Broth – Sipping mineral rich homemade or quality store-bought bone broth aids digestion and reduces intestinal permeability underlying food sensitivities. You may want to ease into drinking straight bone broth. I thought I could just treat it like a soup I could chug, but no, no I could not.

Consider Probiotic Supplements – Capsule formulas with diverse bacterial strains help restore harmony. Those containing Saccharomyces Boulardii show particular cognitive benefit. Start slowly.

LIMIT ANTIBIOTICS – While medically necessary sometimes, antibiotics disrupt delicate gut ecology. Always follow with a course of probiotics.

Manage Stress – Chronic stress depletes beneficial Lactobacillus species. Cultivate rest through meditation, nature, massage, music etc.

Eat Prebiotic Veggies – Asparagus, garlic, onions, leeks provide prebiotic fiber that feeds probiotics and strengthens gut barrier health.

Drink Kombucha – This fermented tea contains probiotics and organic acids benefiting digestion and mental functioning. Check brands for low sugar.

Ask About Testing – If symptoms point to gut/brain imbalance like fatigue, moodiness or food reactions, explore GI specialty testing for bacterial overgrowths, inflammation etc. to guide interventions.

A healthy internal ecosystem strengthens the body-mind connection. Be patient finding the right diet and supplements that optimize both digestion and brain health. Nurture the gut-brain bridge.

The Blessing of Home Cooking

Amidst hectic schedules, it's tempting to rely on takeout, delivery, and packaged snacks instead of home cooked fare. But convenient does not always mean healthy, especially for partners challenged by PCOS and ADHD. Home cooking nourishes in more ways than one.

Control Ingredients – You customize recipes to avoid personal trigger ingredients and boost nutrients needed. No hidden risks.

Manage Portions – Home plated meals make it easier to practice proper portion sizes instead of overdoing restaurant servings.

Save Money – Takeout and ready-made snacks burn through a grocery budget fast. Home cooking provides more nutrition per dollar spent.

Reduce Food Reactions – A cleaner diet nixing additives may lessen sensitivities aggravated by restaurant fare.

Invite Creativity – Cooking at home allows improvisation and recipe experimentation catered to your tastes.

Set Healthy Defaults – When you control the kitchen, ingredients on hand naturally steer you toward better choices instead of packaged snacks.

Build Bonds – Shared meal preparation becomes quality bonding time together filled with conversation.

Practice Mindfulness – Cooking with intention cultivates being more present in the moment versus quick fast food meals.

Teach Life Skills – Passing down recipes and cooking wisdom empowers your partner with knowledge to use for life.

During a time when I was working two jobs, we resorted to meal services such as Hello Fresh to just drop a box of meals on our doorstep once a week. It freed up a lot of time, and the meals were nutritious and portioned for two people. If time is at a premium, I recommended services like this, even for a few nights per week.

While occasional takeout provides relief from meal monotony, make most meals at home the norm. View time in the kitchen not as a chore but an opportunity to work as a team nourishing your bodies and relationship.

Cultivating a Nourishing partnership

More than simply fueling our bodies, meals offer sacred space to nourish bonds and intimacy. A spirit of collaboration, patience and lightheartedness allows couples to harmonize differing needs into a mutually supportive nutrition plan.

Communicate Openly – Have ongoing check-ins about what diet tweaks alleviate or aggravate your respective symptoms so you can adapt menus accordingly.

Surrender Control – If your partner needs to modify diet in ways unlike your own, release rigid expectations. Respect differences.

Make Requests Lovingly – Don't demand dietary changes. Kindly share your preferences and sensitivities and allow your partner space to integrate that insight.

Meal Plan Together – Invite your partner into menu planning in an egalitarian way. Cook together frequently to demystify any new foods.

Allow Flexibility – Don't mandate rigid rules. Grace allows for occasional indulgences, spontaneity, and imperfection.

Focus on Adding in – Emphasize incorporating more nutritional choices into diet instead of just listing restrictions.

Discuss Supplements – Check with your healthcare providers about supplements that foster optimal wellbeing for your respective conditions and relationship. Probiotics, omega-3s, B vitamins, vitamin D, magnesium and more play key roles.

Keep Learning – Continually educate yourselves on emerging nutrition science for both disorders. But don't get overwhelmed implementing everything at once.

Outsource If Needed – If differences feel too frustrating to navigate in-house, seek guidance from a nutrition therapist experienced in both PCOS and ADHD.

Strategic Fasting

Intermittent fasting, meaning periods of deliberately skipping meals, carefully implemented can assist metabolic and brain health for some. But useless done excessively or incorrectly. Approach with caution.

Gradual Introduction - Start by slowly extending overnight fasts to 14-16 hours by pushing breakfast back a bit. Allow the body to adapt before trying full day fasts.

Monitor Blood Sugar - Test glucose levels to ensure they remain stable. Break fast immediately if dizzy, shaky or unfocused. Fasting shouldn't impair function.

Stay Hydrated - Drink ample water and herbal tea during fasts. Dehydration stresses the body.

Note Menstrual Changes - Severe calorie restriction can disrupt ovulation. Track cycle regularity.

Supplement Wisely - Take electrolytes, calcium, iron and B vitamins if fasting for over 16 hours to prevent deficiencies. Discuss with your doctor.

Break Fast Right - Reintroduce food gently focusing on protein, healthy fat and fiber. Don't binge processed carbs and sugar which spike insulin.

Adjust Medications - Consult prescribing doctor about medication timing when fasting. Some doses may need adjusting.

Avoid Daily Fasting - One or two planned fasts weekly works better long term than daily restriction which takes drastic toll.

Listen to Your Body - Discontinue fasting if experiencing headaches, orthostatic hypotension, gut issues, sleep disruption, mood changes or worsening of symptoms.

While fasting works for some, it can easily become counterproductive if taken too far. Proceed with ample education and caution.

The Balancing Act

Finding the optimal dietary formula challenges all partnerships. Patience through trial and error lets you learn how food sensitively shapes both your bodies and relationship. Each phase will require slight recalibration as needs evolve.

Focus on consistently cultivating the foundational pillars: minimally processed wholesome foods, balanced macronutrients, hydration and strategic supplementation. From there, tailor and tweak with care. There's no perfect one size fits all approach – just progress through partnership.

Nourish each other by sharing in both the cooking and companionship. Explore new flavors together. Allow slip ups without judgement. As you each feel increasingly vibrant, you'll develop trust in the method. While the path meanders, your love nourishes the journey.

Communication is Key: Effective Dialogues in Dual Diagnosis Relationships

Open communication provides the foundation for any healthy relationship. However, chronic conditions like PCOS and ADHD can strain connections if partners lack tools tailored to their challenges. When hormones, distractions, impulses, and sensitivities heighten, good intentions get lost in translation.

With mutual compassion, you can learn new dialoguing strategies to enhance understanding. Share your worlds thoughtfully. Listen without judging. Find wisdom in every misunderstanding. Communication is the bridge across any divide when built with care.

Managing Miscommunications

Even in the most conscious relationships, miscommunications inevitably occur. The inherent social and focus challenges those with ADHD face paired with the mood volatility of PCOS amplify misunderstandings. A minor slight you'd likely let roll off your back may wound your partner deeply.

Rather than resenting frequent clarifying, approach exchanges with more listening and less reacting. Often a simple "Say more about what you mean" unveils the true source of hurt. Your partner then feels safe to share vulnerabilities when met with open curiosity, not hasty judgment.

Script flip self-talk also helps prevent reacting defensively. Suppose you snap back thoughtlessly in the heat of tension. Catch yourself, take a breath, and respond again through your partner's perspective - "I can imagine how my tone just now came across as critical and uncaring making you feel unappreciated. I apologize. How can I explain my intent more sensitively?"

Stepping into your partner's experience breeds compassion and a chance to repair rifts before they widen. Healing any disconnection begins with expressing empathy about how she may perceive your words/actions before defending intent. Never dismiss her feelings as irrational or misinterpretations. Seek to understand first.

Challenges will arise, but through openness, you become more skilled navigating misunderstandings in the spirit of "us versus the problem" rather than combative blaming. Communication, when rooted in mutual care, builds trust to weather any storm.

Finding Emotional Safety

Every couple needs a sense of emotional safety in order to take interpersonal risks, be vulnerable and handle conflict maturely. However, the moodiness accompanying PCOS paired with rejection sensitivity inherent in ADHD makes it extra vital. When your partner feels securely cherished by you, it helps counteract overreactivity.

Reflect on whether your current communication patterns foster security:

- Do you insult, roll your eyes, or talk over one another? Swearing and sarcasm signal disrespect.

- Does only one partner's perspective feel valued in disagreements? Equality nurtures safety.

- Do you make caustic remarks disguised as "jokes"? Humor should never shame.

- Do you share grievances about your partner with friends to garner agreement? Venting breeds distance.

- Does defensiveness shut down productive conversations? Listen more, defend less.

- Do you make critical generalized statements like "you always..." or "you never..."? Avoid gross exaggerations.

- Do arguments consistently rehash the same unresolved issues? Seek mediation help if needed.

Now envision how safe communication might look:

- Making time and space for deep sharing where you each feel heard

- Remaining attuned to body language and asking what emotions underlie words

- Giving compliments that reinforce positive qualities and actions

- Using gentle "I feel" statements instead of accusations

- Validating each other's differing needs and perspectives

- Expressing appreciation for efforts made, however imperfect

- Assuming positive intent even when impact was negative

Feeling safe to disclose inner struggles and emotions enables connection. Help your partner open up by ensuring consistent care in your words and responses. Foster a sanctuary where her most tender parts feel welcomed, not judged.

Communicating Through Conflict

In times of tension, our trauma wounds and protective parts readily hijack poised responses. But with skill, conflict can become an avenue for intimacy, not destruction. Some strategies to keep discussions solution-focused:

Time It Thoughtfully – Avoid raising grievances when sleep deprived, hungry, rushed or during PMS cycles when extra irritable. Set time aside to thoughtfully process serious issues.

Define The Issue – Clarify the exact topic at hand. Don't dredge up every petty annoyance. Stick to one resolvable grievance.

Take Turns Speaking – Share your perspective one at a time without interrupting. Feel fully heard before reacting. Misunderstandings surface when we talk over one another.

Use "I Statements" – Discuss how you feel using I not you. "I felt worried and abandoned when you didn't call." It reduces defensiveness.

Listen To Understand – Rather than thinking of counterarguments while your partner talks, listen intently. Reflect her feelings back to ensure you fully grasp them.

Find Common Ground – Connect on mutual hopes underlying contrary stances. "We both want more quality time together. Let's brainstorm ideas."

Take Responsibility – Own your part in the conflict as a springboard for resolution. Change starts within.

Propose Compromises – Be willing to meet halfway. Rigidity ensures both parties' needs stay unmet.

Agree To Disagree - Not every difference requires resolution. Sometimes respectfully accepting certain disagreements grants freedom.

Forgive Quickly – Don't punish your partner repeatedly for mistakes addressed. Set a clean slate for fresh starts.

Approach discord as an opportunity to learn and expand - about your partner's inner world and the dynamics needing nurturing between you. Tensions remind us where we must grow next. Let conflicts cultivate understanding.

Sensitive Subjects: Talking About Sex and Intimacy

Sexual and intimacy challenges rank among the most sensitive subjects for couples managing PCOS and ADHD to navigate. When hormone imbalances lower libido and ADHD distractibility disrupts focus, these core connective acts feel threatened. However, avoiding the topic worsens the wedge between you. Opening courageous conversations around intimacy issues fosters healing.

Pick moments to discuss when you're both feeling open and centered. Use gentle "I statements" to share your experience. "I've noticed I'm often left feeling emotionally as well as physically disconnected when we're intimate because your mind seems preoccupied. Help me understand what that's about."

Listen without judgment as your partner unpacks her struggles around libido or satisfaction. Discuss with an openness to learn not accuse. Share requests for what nourishing intimacy requires from your end. "More relaxing touch throughout the week outside the bedroom would help me feel closer even if sex is less frequent."

Brainstorm together creative solutions that honor both your needs – from sensual activities that don't require penetrative sex to medications that may help override distraction tendencies. Sex and closeness may look different than your expectations. Prioritize emotional intimacy first.

If past resentments still feel unresolved, seeking counseling with a specialist in sexual issues provides great value. Therapeutic perspective helps heal fundamental disconnects. When your loving bond feels securely nurtured in and outside the bedroom through mutual care, intimacy naturally flows.

Communicating With Compassion

Ultimately, compassion and assuming positive intent creates the safety net for weathering any conversation's ebbs and flows. You both want to feel heard and understood, even if misunderstandings sometimes obstruct direct paths.

When communication gets tricky, reflect on how past pain and lifelong social struggles shape your partner's reactions. With empathy and patience, you can unravel even the most tangled discussions. Phrases like "Help me understand where you're coming from" open doors.

Of course your feelings deserve equal consideration. Voice them, but without indictments or contempt. Use language emphasizing mutual partnership, not power leverage. Promote growth, not guilt.

Through openness, mindfulness and good faith, every difficult dialogue strengthens understanding of the beautiful complex beings you both are. What grace it takes at times – but it's the very currency of love.

Cultivating Constructive Conversations

Intentional, constructive communication doesn't just happen. It requires structure promoting safety. Some techniques to try:

Schedule Talk Time – Set recurring times to connect without distractions. Turn off devices, remove clutter, make eye contact. Priority breeds meaning.

Practice Mindful Listening – When your partner speaks, focus fully on comprehending. Minimize planning rebuttals. Let go of other thoughts. Value presence.

Take Breaks If Needed - If tensions heighten, pause the discussion until calm. Leave and self-soothe, then reunite with good faith.

Speak Your Feelings – Even difficult emotions deserve airing in measured tones. Bottling up breeds distance. Release feelings appropriately.

Find Compromise – Insisting on singular stances creates gridlock. Brainstorm solutions honoring each person's needs in balance.

Express Appreciation – Verbalizing gratitude for your partner's efforts, time, and care keeps perspective positive.

Agree On Next Steps – End conversations on action plans for change to prevent lingering ambiguity. Then summarize progress at next talk time.

Accentuate The Positive – Before critiquing negatives, share appreciations and affection. Praise reinforces desired behaviors.

Learn Repair Skills – Amends require reflecting how your actions impacted your partner, sincerely apologizing, asking how to remedy hurt, and outlining behavior change.

When Necessary, Seek Counseling – If chronic conflict plagues discussions, an objective therapist facilitates communication breakthroughs.

Tools like non-violent communication, radical listening, and conflict resolution offer great resources. But lasting growth comes through daily patience, empathy and mutual responsibility.

Keep investing – understanding is the greatest intimacy.

Embracing Nonverbal Cues

Beyond spoken words, the nonverbal dimensions of communication impart deeper messages. Be mindful of the tones, gazes, and body language grounding your exchanges. Aligning nonverbal and verbal creates safety and synchronicity.

Facial Expressions – Ensure your expressions match your words. Smiling, warm eye contact and affirmative head nods reinforce affection.

Physical Touch – Shared oxytocin from handholding, embracing, massage and skin contact soothes and connects. Savor non-sexual physical closeness.

Tone of Voice – Even if words are kind, a tense harsh voice conveys underlying feelings. Keep volume soft and speech warm.

Energy Level – Match your partner's energy when possible by reading vitality signals. Modulate your animation to avoid under or overstimulation.

Body Positioning – Sitting angled toward your partner facing each other signals engagement. Crossed arms and distracted glances unconsciously distance.

Comfort Zone – Note if your proximity helps your partner feel enveloped or overcrowded. Give space or draw nearer as needed.

Timing – Be aware of optimal timing to initiate conversations based on your partner's natural cycles. Mornings may allow more focus than latenights when overtaxed.

Restorative Touch – Offer nurturing physical affection like hand massages or foot rubs to companion difficult discussions and signal caring.

Meditative Embrace – Hug, cuddle or sit wrapped in silence allowing the shared spiritual nourishment to transcend words. Just be together.

Nonverbal communication expresses emotions and intentions beyond vocabulary. By honoring the silent signals, your bonds continue fortifying.

Sexual Well-being: Understanding the Impact of PCOS on Intimacy

Nurturing a satisfying sex life proves challenging for many couples. But when polycystic ovary syndrome enters the bedroom, additional obstacles arise. Between hormone-related libido fluctuations, insulin-driven weight gain, and conception worries, PCOS profoundly impacts women's sexual self-image and functioning.

As a caring partner, your support can be instrumental in buffering these intimacy struggles. Boost your knowledge of common concerns. Help alleviate shame. Prioritize emotional connection. Bring creativity, playfulness and patience under the sheets. While PCOS may recalibrate your love life, trust it can also deepen your bond if navigated with care.

Hormones and Libido: Irregularity and Unpredictability

Female sexual desire involves an intricate dance of hormones. Estrogen energizes libido while progesterone calms it. Ensuring proper balances across the menstrual cycle typically allows spontaneous and rewarding intimacy. However, the hormone havoc PCOS wreaks disrupts this ebb and flow.

Many women with PCOS report they can never predict when their body will be "in the mood". Sex drive peaks and plummets randomly, not aligning with cycle phases. Others describe extended low libido periods interrupted by short-lived ravenous urges. This irregularity and unpredictability bewilders partners.

Rather than shaming your loved one as moody or depriving, recognize how PCOS hijacks hormones dictating desire outside her control. She likely feels equally frustrated by the sexual catch-22s. Track patterns together with patience. Help facilitate intimacy during her passionate peaks while offering closeness without pressure in troughs. Reassure her this symptom spectrum is normal for PCOS, not deficient desire.

Also investigate potential medication influences. Certain treatments like oral contraceptives and anti-androgens alter testosterone levels affecting arousal. Discuss options with her prescriber. While struggling with unpredictable desire breeds distress, your empathy and creativity can temper effects.

Mood Impacts: Irritability, Depression and Anxiety's Influence

In addition to erratic hormones undermining consistent sexual engagement, negative mood states also commonly quash libido for women with PCOS. The inherent metabolic and endocrine disruptions often breed conditions like clinical depression, anxiety, poor body image, sleep disturbances, chronic pain and fatigue – all desire deterrents.

Coping with these mood consequences alone breeds isolation. Your partner may feel you couldn't possibly understand depths of her anguish and disengagement. But your listening ear helps shoulder the load. Check in frequently about her mood patterns:

"How are you feeling emotionally lately with all the PCOS anxiety and depression?"

"It seems like you've been really sad and distant this week during a hormone crash. How can I be supportive when that hits?"

"I know intimacy is hard when you're fighting this low mood. But I'm here for comfort and closeness in any way."

If depressive or anxious states persist, delicately suggest seeking therapy and medical support. Emphasize you view it as another form of healthcare, not personal failure. If she consents to couples counseling, therapists can impart techniques preventing bedroom disconnects and fostering emotional intimacy when libido lags.

Most importantly, never take mood-related sexual disinterest personally. Hold space for the darkness, so light returns.

Weight Struggles and Body Shame

PCOS frequently brings with it rapid weight gain and inability to shed pounds easily. Even slender women with PCOS often develop new excess weight, facial hair, acne and difficulty toning from metabolic disruptions. The physical changes profoundly affect feminine identity and self-image.

Your partner may feel self-conscious and embarrassed undressing with you, avoiding intimacy that highlights perceived flaws. Sometimes adopting rigid diet and exercise regimens to forcecorrect "problem areas" worsens the dysmorphic obsession. She may project anger about her body onto you.

Combat the distorted lens poor self-image casts by consistently reinforcing your eyes perceive her as beautiful and desirable as ever. Affirm her identity as far more than just physical looks. Compliment small changes she makes toward better self-care, like nutritious meals or brief workouts, reminding her you're partners in long-term progress.

If these strategies aren't enough to conquer body shame, explore pathways like counseling or support groups to unpack the inner critic's powerful hold. But never minimize insecurities fueled by PCOS weight shifts and hypervigilance. Help your partner define herself on her own terms, not society's.

Conception Worries: Stress of Infertility

Many couples managing PCOS brace for difficulties conceiving given irregular ovulation challenges. Even those not yet trying to get pregnant may dread future infertility blows down the line. In fact, anxiety around reproductive ability impacts libido and sensual dynamics long before actively attempting to conceive.

Make space for your partner to voice fertility worries without minimizing them or jumping to problem-solving mode. Listen closely:

"I can only imagine how overwhelming the thought of infertility must feel. It makes total sense you feel preemptive sadness about that."

"Just know that no matter what challenges we may eventually face trying to conceive, we'll tackle them together. This doesn't change how much I love you and want to be with you in life."

"I understand your despair. At the same time, plenty of women with PCOS ultimately conceive even if it takes more time. And we have options."

Take any pressure off your sexual relationship "performing" the job of conception. There are many paths to parenthood. Instead nurture intimacy just for the sake of pleasure, play, and connection in the moment. When sex carries a duty, it becomes a chore. Protect your physical bond by keeping it joyful.

Vaginal Dryness and Painful Sex

Certain PCOS symptoms also create physical discomfort during intercourse leading many couples to avoid sex. Vaginal dryness results from low estrogen combined with obesity. Insulin resistance promotes yeast overgrowth and related discharge/irritation as well. PCOS-linked conditions like endometriosis also cause pelvic muscle spasms and pain.

Open communication allows you to be thoughtful lovers, tuning into signals that penetration feels uncomfortable or impossible without shaming your partner's symptoms:

"Just tell me what feels good tonight. We can focus just on foreplay and external stimulation."

"Let me know if you get any pinching or tightness and we can switch positions or grab the lubricant."

"There are still so many ways we can enjoy physical closeness and take the focus off intercourse. I'm happy just cuddling and holding you."

Foremost, let your partner guide the pace and activities without taking physical limitations personally. Prioritize sensual variety, lubrication, responsive feedback, and unconditional acceptance. Move slowly with caresses, kisses, and massage building arousal and relaxation.

Make intimacy pleasurable, not goal oriented.

Discuss medical interventions like prescription estrogen creams, pelvic floor therapy, or pain medications with her healthcare provider as needed. But meanwhile, let comfort and creativity steer your encounters.

Holistic Approaches: Lifestyle, Diet, Movement and Mindset

While PCOS poses formidable intimacy obstacles, certain holistic measures can help mitigate challenges and reboot libido:

Target exercise – Find regular sensual movement she enjoys like dancing, yoga, Pilates. Anything increasing circulation, endorphins and flexibility aids arousal.

Eat clean – An anti-inflammatory whole foods diet improves hormone balance and body image perceptions. Stay hydrated and minimize alcohol.

Destress life – Make time for relaxing bonding activities without outside stressors. Give space for self-care rituals like baths, massages, nature walks.

Manage medications – Explore adjusting formulations if BC pills, anti-androgens or antidepressants seem to blunt desire. Discuss with her provider.

Supplement strategically – Tribulus, shatavari, maca, zinc and vitamin D support sexual health and hormones when used carefully under medical guidance.

Practice self-love – Encourage exploring her sensual sides alone through music, fantasies, and toys. Developing sexual self-awareness translates to shared intimacy. Even manually stimulating her brings you closer sexually.

Reframe mindset – Release goal-driven attitudes around arousal and orgasm. Instead savor sensation and emotional union.

Try alternatives – When intercourse proves impossible, engage sensually through gentle erotic touch, kissing, fantasy sharing, bathing together, oral pleasures, or adult toys.

A vow of loving patience and teamwork braces you through all PCOS may bring to your intimate life. While some days limitations feel discouraging, intimacy fluctuates. Trust in the ebb and flow, just as in any aspect of lifelong partnership.

Cultivating Sexual and Emotional Intimacy

While PCOS potentially affects the mechanics of sex, the deeper solutions address nurturing intimacy foundations. Truly secure and satisfying sensual relating stems from sustained emotional connection inside and outside the bedroom.

Don't put all pressure solely on overtly sexual exchanges which may feel vulnerable and emotionally loaded for your partner when struggling with self-confidence, hormones, and pain. Instead focus daily attention on building trust, familiarity and affection through subtle gestures:

- Offer relaxing massages without expectation of intercourse after.

- Cuddle, kiss, and be affectionate at non-sexual times just expressing closeness.

- Cook a romantic meal together then slow dance in the kitchen.

- Exchange love letters about cherished memories and future dreams.

- Hold hands during walks or drives. Maintain eye contact when conversing.

- Give small thoughtful gifts like flowers or sweet notes expressing appreciation.

- Flirt playfully throughout the day via texts, winks across the room, inside jokes.

- Discuss favorite sensual memories, fantasies, and desires openly outside pressured moments.

As your shared sense of safety, care, tenderness, and mutual fulfillment strengthens, sexual flow naturally follows. But don't expect this overnight, especially when PCOS and confidence struggles are at play. Healing happens gradually through consistency. Plant seeds of devotion – they'll bear fruits in time.

When to Seek Sex Therapy

If PCOS severely disrupts your sex life or breeds relationship discord, seeking guidance from a qualified sex therapist or counselor provides immense value. Specialists offer tools to overcome obstacles and reconnect intimately.

Some signs it may be time to get support:

- Ongoing tension, arguments or avoidance around sex

- Months of infrequent intimacy with no apparent medical cause

- Strong shame or inadequacy associated with sexual interactions

- Persisting uncomfortable mechanics or pain during sex

- Sudden onset of emotional detachment or hostility between partners

- Suspicions of cheating or withdrawal due to needs unmet

- One partner exhibiting consistently higher libido straining the bond

- Persistent body image anxieties killing the sensual mood

- Trauma history impairing ability to be present and vulnerable during sex

With expert help, you'll gain insights into your sexual patterns and blocks. Exercises build sensual confidence and tuned-in touch. Most importantly, counseling fortifies your intimate friendship and sense of safety sharing your whole selves.

If intimacy issues ever threaten the heartbeat of your partnership, remember – help is available. You must both feel cherished on all levels for the foundation to thrive. With radical compassion and willingness, PCOS can deepen your connection, not derail it.

Honoring Her Resilience and Yours

Finally, I encourage you to recognize your partner's incredible sensual resilience despite obstacles PCOS may interject. Forge ahead with admiration, not frustration. Likewise, acknowledge your own reservoirs of patience and commitment nurturing your bond through all seasons. You are both the very definitions of brave, passionate lovers.

Remember, an intimate relationship stands upon far more than physical expression alone, though that holds importance too. Your souls, hopes, values, and dreams weave the tapestry – sexuality just one of many colorful threads. When you approach sex as a celebration of lifelong love, it transforms in meaning.

Cherish your partner and the relationship you've manifested. Each day, find small sincere ways to honor the monumental gift true intimacy represents. Through PCOS and in joy, you walk forward hand in hand.

Embracing the Hyperfocus: Utilizing ADHD Strengths in Daily Life

While attention deficits cause very real problems for those with ADHD, there is an incredible gift hiding in the neurodiversity of their minds: hyperfocus. When passionately engaged in activities of interest, your partner likely achieves flow states of deep concentration and productivity — what ADHD communities fondly call hyperfocus.

However, outside observers often misperceive hyperfocus as simply the ability to focus, rather than the intensified fixation unique to ADHD minds. In truth, hyperfocus represents both blessing and curse. When harnessed strategically, it allows partners with ADHD to flourish creatively and tap genius states. Let's explore how to embrace hyperfocus as a relationship superpower.

Defining the Phenomenon

Hyperfocus describes an enhanced state of distraction-free flow, energy and absorption experienced by those with ADHD around tasks captivating their interests. Studies estimate 70-80% of people with ADHD report frequent hyperfocus activation. It represents a key advantage of their neurotype.

Unlike the transient focus neurotypicals exert through effort, hyperfocus grants an immersive tunnel vision making all else around melt away. Partners describe losing all sense of time and place for hours or even days when engrossed in stimulating projects. The outside world ceases to exist.

However, once the captivating activity ends, awareness of priorities neglected during the hyperfocus episode comes flooding back. Time blindness sets in. While the project at hand reached new heights, responsibilities and relationships may have suffered unintended neglect.

Hyperfocus is not simply the ability to pay attention or buckle down on demand. It occurs involuntarily based on intrinsic rewards, not external pressures. Partners with ADHD often cannot focus consistently on tasks they find boring or draining regardless of incentives. But give them freedom pursuing passions, and incredible magic unfolds.

Drivers and Characteristics

What exactly turns on the switch of hyperfocus? Certain conditions activate and maximize this state of creative flow:

- Autonomy over focus area without structured rules

- High interest level based on novelty and curiosity

- Immediate feedback loops spurring dopamine

- Immersive sensory environment removing distractions

- Scope requiring imagination and interdisciplinary skills

Hyperfocus commonly occurs while learning new instruments, playing video games, developing computer applications, painting, writing fiction, building models, playing sports, analyzing data, perfecting a recipe — any activity blissfully captivating.

Outward signs of hyperfocus include:

- Loss of awareness of time passing

- Delayed responsiveness to stimuli like hunger, thirst, fatigue

- Impatience with external interruptions

- Not hearing others calling their name

- Irritability when pulled from task prematurely

- Need for sensory dimming like noise cancelling headphones

- Intense energy and animation while engrossed

By recognizing your partner's hyperfocus "tells", you can better avoid disruption during these fruitful phases. Have needs-related discussions planned around predictable windows of fixation. Protect the gift of their vast imagination and creativity.

Harnessing Hyperfocus as an Asset

Rather than resenting episodes of intense absorption, reframe your partner's hyperfocus as an asset to nurture. Help identify meaningful avenues through work, hobbies, and volunteer roles to direct hyperfocus productivity.

When employed purposefully, hyperfocus grants partners with ADHD ability to:

- Master skills through obsessive quality practice

- Immerse in creative arts like writing, music, handicrafts

- Innovate novel approaches to problems

- Excel in STEM fields through pattern recognition

- Research topics thoroughly delving into granular details

- Enter visionary states breeding groundbreaking ideas

- Accomplish in days or hours intensive projects that may take teammates weeks

By channeling passions into career and personal outlets, hyperfocus results in new business ventures, novels written, record times achieved, inventions built, causes championed. Rather than lamenting distractions, celebrate the depths of dedication.

You can lovingly help your partner identify optimal hyperfocus domains through questions like:

"What topics could you explore for hours losing track of everything else?"

"When have you experienced being so creatively in the zone that amazing results occurred?"

"What activities make you feel energized and fulfilled for their own sake?"

Then collaborate designing structures maximizing hyperfocus benefits: crafting home offices minimizing distractions, leveraging passions in career paths, scheduling creative time.

With some curation, hyperfocus becomes an incredible relationship gift — the power of presence transformed into achievements nurturing you both.

Strategies for Everyday Functioning

Beyond pursuing passions, your partner can also apply hyperfocus strategically to everyday responsibilities. Mundane tasks may never captivate like artistic endeavors. However, certain techniques lend focus:

- Break larger goals into mini-quests with measurable progress providing dopamine spurts.

- Gamify schedules by tracking productivity stats and creating rewards for consistency.

- Pair boring tasks with beloved music, snacks, or tactile toys creating positive associations.

- Verbally narrate workflow step-by-step to maintain focus momentum.

- Visually chart progress through wall calendars, checklists, and process flows.

- Timebox periods for household chores, exercise, and work projects balancing hyperfocus.

- Batch similar tasks together in themed blocks versus context switching.

- Compete against personal bests to harness competitive drive.

- Creatively multitask by integrating physical activity into learning.

You can also kindly help minimize external disruptions during designated focus blocks. Offer guarding space as a gift.

The motivation must arise within, but you can scaffold conditions optimizing hyperfocus for real world responsibilities. With innovation, even mundane tasks become more achievable.

Preventing Negative Impacts

Without boundaries, hyperfocus tendencies present challenges like:

- Forgetting to eat, sleep, or attend to hygiene while absorbed

- Avoiding unappealing tasks despite consequences

- Becoming so engrossed in personal projects that relationships, family duties, and work suffer

- Struggling to transition focus when needed resulting in tardiness

- Allowing the quick rewards of gaming or social media to dominate free time

- Feeling depressed when passion projects conclude

You can lovingly collaborate on structures protecting against hyperfocus pitfalls:

- Ring reminder alarms for breaks, meals, and sleep during absorption spells.

- Institute "no electronics" family time protecting quality bonding.

- Set aside specific days for mundane tasks like cleaning to prevent neglect.

- Help redirect fixation when responsibilities require immediate attention.

- Encourage savoring the journey of creativity, not just final outcomes.

- Schedule incremental progress on long-term goals for sustainable pacing.

Without judgment, find ways to celebrate hyperfocus talents while establishing healthy boundaries. With compassion, channel its power productively.

Embracing Your Partner's Neurological Gifts

Rather than viewing your partner's hyperfocus as problematic intensity, recognize it as an incredible neurological gift. Their capacity for absolute presence and creative fixation reveals the beauty of their ADHD minds. Help foster activities eliciting flow. Protect space for imagination. Ask about passion projects with genuine wonder.

No doubt hyperfocus has both light and shadow sides like any trait. But by leaning into strengths, you empower your partner to curate career, hobbies, and habits leveraging motivational superpowers.

ADHD wiring confers unique genius when nurtured well. Your role is helping rewrite limiting narratives about distraction and inability. Loving partners reflect back talents waiting to be recognized. When you celebrate hyperfocus, you honor the spirited creator residing in your beloved's soul.

Body Image & Self-Esteem: Building Confidence Together

Partners grappling with the simultaneous effects of PCOS and ADHD often confront harsh struggles with body image and self-worth. Weight fluctuations, hormonal changes, focus challenges, and societal stigma batter self-confidence in insidious ways. As a loving partner, you hold tremendous power to lift shame and build genuine self-acceptance. With consistent love mirrored back, she can learn to embrace imperfection and recognize her worth. Let's explore thoughtful strategies for nurturing self-esteem and positive embodiment together.

Impacts of PCOS on Body Image and Self-Perception

Polycystic ovary syndrome profoundly shapes physical appearance and self-concept. Hormone-driven symptoms like rapid weight gain, excess hair growth, severe acne, and alopecia all negatively impact women's bodily experience. Genetic factors beyond their control swiftly alter contour and complexion.

Simultaneously, related metabolic issues like insulin resistance, inflammation, and fatigue sap motivation needed for self-care. Exercise and healthy meal prep become monumental tasks when just getting through daily obligations feels overwhelming. This compounds frustrations about weight.

Outwardly, society and media perpetuate narrow beauty ideals valuing thinness and flawless complexions. Your partner compares herself feeling inadequate. Inwardly, distorted body image sinks self-worth. She may fixate on perceived imperfections that you barely notice.

While you see only her beauty, she dwells on exaggerating "problems"— belly pooch, thinning hair, skin blemishes, cellulite dimples. Any small aesthetic change signifies failure because her sense of empowerment and acceptance got entangled with physical looks molded by illness.

Have compassion realizing comments about diet, exercise, and cosmetic fixes likely stem from profound insecurity, not vanity. Her self-concept is under siege. Lift her up with consistent messages about inherent worth beyond appearance. Help redefine beauty as confidence shining through.

ADHD Symptoms Undermining Self-Esteem

Alongside PCOS struggles, ADHD symptoms also deliver blows to self-image. Chronic disorganization, forgetfulness, missed deadlines, and impulsive choices easily get interpreted as personal failings and character flaws. Your partner berates herself rather than recognizing neurological origins.

ADHD-related social and learning struggles also breed self-blame. She may carry embarrassment about needing more time on tasks, getting overstimulated easily, or missing social cues others intuit. Childhood stigma sticks as shame haunting adult self-perception.

Additionally, RSD (rejection sensitive dysphoria) common with ADHD magnifies perceptions of failure and judgement from you and others. Casual critiques cut deep, confirming secret anxieties about inadequacy. Unsupportive partners amplify negative core beliefs.

Your encouraging presence provides a secure base protecting against distortions. Affirm her worth comes from far more than productivity levels, social polish, or test scores. Instill that messiness, mistakes, and quirks make her beautifully human. Help reframe ADHD differences as diversity, not deficiencies.

Guide her from measuring self-value against unrealistic standards. What truly matters are relationships nurtured, passions pursued, values lived. Anchor her in these truths.

Cultivating Body Positivity and Self-Love

Shifting from toxic inner voices to compassionate self-talk requires diligent practice. Help your partner build awareness of negative patterns and consistently counter with loving wisdom.

Notice judgments – Ask her to pause when hearing self-criticism arise and reflect: "If a friend spoke about herself this harshly, how would I respond?" Visualizing it as bullying a loved one exposes its cruelty.

Identify roots – Explore together where messages like "I'm lazy and ugly" originated. Was it a parent, ex, media? Unpack their biases versus truths. Arm her against old wounds hijacking self-perception.

Rewrite stories – Guide her to start journaling affirmations daily. Record positive qualities, talents, and spiritual essence until the supportive narrative drowns out the harsh one.

Focus on character – Compliment admirable traits like kindness, integrity, and perseverance. Remind her embodiments of wisdom, wit, and care define her, not temporary looks.

Praise self-care – Cheer small daily wellness habits like nutritious meals, brief walks, yoga stretches, meditation, and early bedtimes. Link self-love to actions, not just appearance.

Confront comparisons – When she fixates on flaws versus others' perfection, ask "Would you speak about your cherished friends like this?" Comparisons say more about our self-judgment than others' worth.

Allow imperfection – Help release the need to be flawless. Flaws are what make us beautifully human, loved for authenticity. Model self-acceptance out loud through lighthearted humor about your own "flaws".

Surround with support – Introduce body positive books, podcasts, counselors, and support groups conveying her reflections of inadequacy are distorted, not reality. Health is about nourishment and caring for needs, not chasing ideals.

Keep aligning her eyes with truth – she is whole and worthy beyond any transient physical changes or mental struggles. Her light deserves to shine.

Cultivating a Team Mindset Around Health

Rather than preaching discipline when your partner's motivation lags, reframe health goals as a collaborative effort. Make wellbeing practices sources of joint support and intimacy versus solitary burdens.

Ask "How can I be helpful as your partner in this?" Tangibly assist with meal plans, workout accountability, scheduling doctor visits, and creating supplements checklists. Handle hurdles as a team.

Compliment every nourishing choice from brief walks to balanced breakfasts. Don't critique "cheat" days. Progress flows from encouragement. Create incentives like massages, dance parties, or fun outings to celebrate milestones.

Focus your concern on how she feels physically and mentally with current lifestyle habits versus judging numeric outcomes. Ask about symptoms, energy levels, self-care practices. Stress you care about her health arising from self-love, not pressure to transform appearance.

Guide her to direct anger at the illnesses, not personal flaws. Say "You're working so hard managing symptoms outside your control. I admire your persistence through the frustration." Validate her efforts.

Most importantly, model balanced self-care and body positive language yourself. As her partner, your actions speak volumes. Don't critique your own body harshly. Make time for activities and nutrition nurturing mental health. Mirror the messages of radical self-acceptance you want reflected back to her.

When wellbeing arises from a space of security, collaboration and compassion, it becomes sustainable. What you water together grows.

Nurturing Sensuality and Body Confidence

As physical intimacy often suffers when bodily changes and insecurities accompany PCOS, gently help your partner reconnect with sensuality in meaningful ways. Don't initiate sex expecting lust to override self-consciousness. Instead try:

- Giving relaxing sensual massages focusing on touch not goal-driven pleasure.

- Sharing a warm bath with candles simply holding one another and gazing into eyes.

- Dancing closely to music in dim lighting. Move and laugh together playfully.

- Exploring calming mindfulness-based sex practices like tantric exercises emphasizing presence.

- Complementing unique aspects of her body you find irresistible. Make sincere compliments about both outer and inner qualities.

- Introducing sex toys or fantasy play inviting low-pressure creativity versus performance pressure.

- Keeping sex intimate interactions private to protect vulnerability. Don't discuss details with outside parties.

- Requesting feedback on touch, positions, and pacing supporting her comfort levels. Follow her lead.

- Encouraging her self-pleasure exploration through music, fantasy, and toys. Sexual self-awareness nurtures partnered intimacy.

- Photographing sensual (but not explicitly sexual) embraces focusing on emotional connection and care.

Cherish your shared sensuality as sacred space for reverent adoration, playfulness, and renewal. Help your partner define pleasure and beauty on her own terms. When body confidence blossoms from within, self-love flourishes.

Supporting Her Style as Self-Expression

Beyond body shape, support your partner finding styles allowing her personality to shine. Avoid pushing rigid gendered fashion norms. Encourage seeing clothing and grooming as avenues for self-expression.

ADHD sensory differences mean certain fabrics and textures that you find comfortable may overstimulate her. Help her tune into cues like itchiness or constriction exacerbating restlessness. Suggest soft natural fibers and adjustable fits allowing freedom of movement.

Similarly, fluctuating symptoms like acne or unwanted hair growth may make committing to complex makeup or hair regimens feel futile or frustrating. Gently assure her barefaced radiance needs no filters. Compliment small grooming habits like skin care routines helping her feel her best. Don't judge messy hair days.

Frame style exploration as playful creativity finding colors, patterns, and silhouettes that spark joy. Shop thrift stores together inventing bold looks on weekends for fun, not just for special events. Photography and fashion magazines inspire expression.

Avoid comments that imply she must correct or conceal perceived flaws. Support body hair removal only if she initiates requests, not from your distaste. Affirm she is beautiful as fully herself, not just when molded to conventions.

Holding Space as Her Confidence Grows

Some days when shame and doubt drag your partner under, simply holding space for her to express darkness without judgment allows catharsis. She feels truly seen, not just placated or dismissed.

Listen closely to understand roots of distress without rushing reassurance or solutions. Reflect her feelings back genuinely so she feels heard:

"It makes so much sense this painful feeling stems from years of carrying stigma about your body. I can't imagine how exhausting and defeating that burden feels."

"You have every right to feel angry and grieving over the way this illness has robbed your vibrancy lately. I know your light is still in there behind the clouds."

As she unloads shame, convey your unconditional love:

"These changes are just what health and aging bring to our temporary physical forms, not your essence. Your spirit always remains beautiful."

"There is absolutely nothing you could look like or be capable of doing that would make me admire or desire you any less. My love reflects your whole being."

By holding space free of judgment when insecurities arise, you help release their grip. She no longer feels compelled to hide struggles from you. Setbacks transform into opportunities for intimacy and growth.

Together, turn shame from a lonely prison into freedom through courageous expression of shadows. Into your safe harbor she can sail the deepest waters.

Body Image & Self-Esteem: Building Confidence Together

Living with chronic health conditions like PCOS and ADHD often deeply affects women's self-image and self-worth. When ongoing symptoms challenge societal beauty ideals and make self-care consistency difficult, insecurities and criticism creep in. As her partner, you hold immense power to nurture positive embodiment and purpose. Build confidence through compassion, not judgment. Help rewrite limiting narratives about her right to joy. Together you can transform struggles into sources of strength.

Healing Her Relationship with Her Body

The metabolic effects accompanying PCOS frequently trigger rapid, unwanted weight gain and make slimming extremely difficult. Excess hair growth and acne often emerge as well. Meanwhile, ADHD related disorganization and impulsiveness sabotage routines promoting fitness and wellbeing.

These physical changes profoundly impact women's body image, as society harshly judges any deviation from conventional attractiveness. As a result, many partners with PCOS/ADHD come to view their bodies as the enemy, something to critique and control. Self-esteem suffers under the never-ending project to fix flaws.

Start by helping your partner separate her body from her identity. Affirm all the non-physical qualities deeply unique and loveable about her – creativity, humor, passions, talents, quirks.

"You are so much more than your appearance, my love." When she sees her true essence as far more than looks, insecurities hold less sway.

Emphasize that her diagnoses don't define her worthiness of self-care. She deserves nourishing food, comfortable clothing, enjoyable movement, and sensuality no matter her size or symptoms. Help make self-care rituals accessible.

Share what you find beautiful about her body and presence. Compliment her personal style and strong limbs capable of activity. Notice small positive changes she implements for herself but may overlook.

Finally, suggest working with a therapist if poor body image hinders joie de vivre. You want your partner embracing her body as an instrument for living, not an ornament for judging. With practice, body neutrality and care replace criticism.

Building Her Self-Confidence and Resilience

Beyond the physical, compromised self-esteem often plagues women managing PCOS and ADHD. They become trapped comparing accomplishments to others instead of appreciating strengths. You can gently help build realistic confidence and purpose.

Reflect on her talents and wing gifts: intense focus when captivated, high perceptiveness, creativity, big picture thinking, passion, humor, charisma. Remind your partner of the unique value she adds simply by being herself.

When she spirals into negative self-talk, provide a loving reality check. Help redirect from unproductive rumination into actions expressing her talents. Enable pursuing dreams.

Share examples of those thriving powerfully with her diagnoses. Neurodiversity allows forging uncommon paths. There are no "normal" benchmarks.

Suggest writing gratitude lists when she feels discouraged - little joys, privileges, or kindnesses she may take for granted when overlooking her own gifts out of scarcity thinking. Gratitude breeds appreciation.

Finally, model self-acceptance about your own perceived shortcomings. You demonstrate how to acknowledge room for growth while speaking kindly to yourself. The more fulfilled you feel in your purpose, the more you can inspire your partner's confidence.

Nurturing Friendships and Community

PCOS and ADHD often cultivate sensitivity and emotional intensity. Without adequate social connection, partners can feel alienated, misunderstood, and overly self-critical. Help your loved one prioritize friendship and community for self-worth resilience.

Support connecting with fellow neurodivergent people through in-person groups, forums, or social media. Shared experiences combat isolation. You don't have to journey alone.

Make time for supportive social outings together and separately. Plan regular video chats over coffee with long-distance friends. Companionship fuels the spirit.

Discuss volunteering for causes tapping into her passions. Contributing strengths boosts confidence and joy.

If she resists socializing due to fatigue or avoidance tendencies, gently encourage small outings. Remind her that spending time with loved ones often energizes.

Ultimately confidence blooms from within through self-love. But tender friendships help reflect inner light. With your encouragement, help your partner surround herself with nurturing community.

Managing The Depression and Anxiety Connection

Women with PCOS and ADHD have significantly higher risks for mood disorders like depression and anxiety compared to the general public. Their symptoms intricately interplay, leading to a vicious bidirectional cycle. Low mood aggravates focus challenges, isolation, and self-neglect, which in turn worsens feelings of emptiness, worthlessness, and worry.

This highly stigmatized mental health trap can profoundly scar self-esteem if inadequately managed. While no fast fixes exist, certain steps make space for healing:

Help your partner recognize symptoms like persistent low mood, lack of enjoyment, changes in sleep and appetite, mental clouding, and suicidal thinking as possible depression requiring support, not personal weakness. You view it just like any other health condition needing treatment.

Collaboratively track triggers, thought patterns and lifestyle factors that seem to worsen or lift moods. Keep an open, non-judgmental dialogue.

Research therapy options together – CBT, DBT, mindfulness approaches – and sit in on initial visits if welcomed. Traditional talk therapy proves inadequate alone.

Encourage journaling, creative expression, physical activity or any healthy outlets providing mental release. Avoid numbing through overeating, gambling, impulsive spending or substance abuse.

Help manage daily functioning with mood-friendly nutrition, prompts to socialize, tools for organization, and reducing unnecessary stress.

Guide your partner in speaking openly with her medical team about significant mood symptoms so medications can be evaluated. Brain chemistry deficits sometimes necessitate pharmaceutical support.

Let your steady belief in her inherent value anchor your partner through stormy mental health setbacks. With professional treatment and lifestyle adjustments, the sun keeps rising. She needn't journey alone.

Protecting Self-Care Time

Women tend to expend energy caring for others while minimizing their own needs. However, those managing the demands of PCOS and ADHD especially require prioritizing self-nourishment to prevent depletion. Help your partner preemptively carve out restorative time.

Track how daily obligations, distractions, saying yes too often, and letting pleasurable outlets lapse breed burnout. Self-care cannot remain the leftovers.

Collaboratively map out a weekly self-care plan balancing socializing, relaxing alone time, creative outlets, household duties, and health habits. Treat this calendar commitment as any serious responsibility not to bump.

Model saying no to added commitments when your plate feels full. Demonstrate openly preserving your own rejuvenation margins amidst busy seasons.

Suggest small daily stress-relieving practices like meditating, diffusing essential oils, keeping a gratitude journal, or sipping tea mindfully. Little rituals compound.

Remind your partner she deserves self-care. Her health conditions make rest emotionally and physically essential, not frivolous. You want to see her nurtured.

Debunk any lingering messaging that self-care is selfish. Pouring into your own cup is what allows giving abundantly to others from an authentically full heart.

By elevating self-nourishment together to the status of necessity rather than luxury, you help your partner build reserves of energy and confidence. Protect that sacred space for her.

Rewriting Limiting Narratives

Finally, reflect on any internalized false narratives stemming from PCOS and ADHD that undermine your partner recognizing her worthiness exactly as she is. Help lovingly rewrite those stories.

If her inner critic says:

"I'm just lazy, unmotivated and can't keep up." → Remind her ADHD is a neurotype, not a choice. Her brain functions differently, not worse. Everyone needs unique environments to thrive.

"I'm incapable of really taking care of my health." → PCOS and ADHD do make consistency extra challenging! Allow imperfection. Progress comes step by step. You're by her side.

"My mood swings make me too much to handle."

→ Validate her experiences as real, not imagined. Her sensitive nervous system is a gift as much as struggle. You signed up for all of her.

"I'll never achieve what normal people do." → Challenging norms is her superpower! She envisions possibilities and brings unconventional gifts to the world. There is no one path to success.

"I don't deserve intimacy when I'm so disconnected from my body." → Every body deserves intimacy, pleasure and care – absolutely including hers as is in this moment, not some imagined ideal.

As her loyal partner, never underestimate your power to rewrite old scripts of self-judgement into ones affirming her wholeness. Your words water the seeds of self-belief she replants daily. Together cultivate confidence through compassion.

Management and Treatment: Medical and Holistic Approaches

Navigating the complex web of lifestyle changes, medications, therapies, and alternative interventions for PCOS and ADHD can feel incredibly overwhelming. It often takes years of trial and error to discover the optimal personal recipe balancing treatments while minimizing side effects and costs. As a supportive partner, you play a key role on this journey of active collaboration and self-advocacy. Let's explore the full range of medical and holistic options to create an integrated plan.

Deciphering Diverse PCOS Treatment Approaches

Given the multifaceted nature of PCOS, an integrative treatment plan tailored to the specific manifestations in each woman works best. Certain lifestyle interventions prove foundational while medications address acute symptoms. Maintaining realistic expectations helps weather the process of finding the right prescriptions and dosages which takes diligent trial and error. Have patience adjusting treatment elements over time as symptoms fluctuate.

Nutrition – An anti-inflammatory whole foods diet rich in plants, lean proteins, healthy fats, and fiber helps regulate weight, insulin response, hormones, and mental health. Those with PCOS are advised to minimize refined carbohydrates, added sugars, and saturated fats which spike blood sugar and inflammation. Targeted supplements like myo-inositol and omega-3s offer additional benefit.

Exercise – Regular physical activity, even light exercise, assists weight management, circulation, pain symptoms, endorphins and energy levels. Any enjoyable, sustainable movement like walking, yoga, Pilates, cycling, dancing etc. boosts health. However, intense workouts excessively stress the body for those with PCOS. Moderate consistent activity proves most beneficial long-term.

Stress Relief – Managing stress through sufficient sleep, social connection, nature time, hobbies, counseling, meditation, massage, and preventive self-care all help control cortisol and inflammatory flares making PCOS worse. Don't underestimate lifestyle's impact.

Hormonal Birth Control – Oral contraceptive pills help regulate periods, protect the endometrium, decrease androgens, and reduce risks of ovarian and endometrial cancer. Various formulations and delivery methods exist to target specific needs. Discuss benefits and side effects of each with her provider.

Androgen Blockers – Medications like spironolactone and finasteride block androgen hormone receptors helping minimize excess facial/body hair, acne, and scalp hair loss from high testosterone. Topical eflornithine cream slows hair growth. Laser hair removal also works for many.

Fertility Treatment – Options range from ovulation induction pills like clomiphene and letrozole to injectable gonadotropins for timed intercourse or IUI to IVF for those with more involved infertility issues. Risks like higher order multiples exist with some fertility medications.

Metabolic Medications – Drugs like metformin improve insulin sensitivity and aid weight loss along with berberine, inositol, and thiazolidinediones. Statins, fibrates, niacin, and omega-3s help normalize cholesterol. Careful monitoring for side effects is essential.

Mental Health Medication – Those with anxiety, depression, OCD, or other mood disorders related to PCOS may benefit from short-term psychiatric medications alongside therapy and self-care. Combination birth control pills can help stabilize mood swings as well.

Anti-Inflammatories – Due to inflammation's role, some benefit from short courses of over-the-counter NSAIDs like ibuprofen to reduce oxidative stress, pain, and endocrine disruption. Always take with food and avoid long-term due to GI risks.

Surgery – Some with severe chronic anovulation and insulin resistance undergo ovarian drilling, a laparoscopic procedure using electrocautery to induce normal ovulation. However, benefits often only last around 6-9 months before other treatments resume. Risks include reduced ovarian reserve.

Complementary Approaches – Alternative medicine options like acupuncture, supplements, myo-inositol, spearmint tea, stress reduction techniques, light therapy, and more show benefit reducing inflammation, regulating cycles, supporting metabolism, and improving mental health. Work with practitioners skilled in integrative women's medicine.

PCOS management works best when combining prescription treatments targeting the most disruptive symptoms with sustainable lifestyle measures addressing root causes. Have reasonable expectations, educate yourself about all options, and regularly evaluate progress and satisfaction.

Navigating Treatments for ADHD in Adulthood

If your partner receives an ADHD diagnosis as an adult, medications often provide the cornerstone for management. But multimodal plans integrating prescription drugs, counseling, brain training tools, and lifestyle balance prove most successful long-term. Patience is key as finding optimal treatments takes months. Let's explore options:

Stimulant Medications – Amphetamines like Adderall and methylphenidate formulations such as Ritalin remain first-line pharmaceutical treatments for ADHD. At proper doses, stimulants reduce hyperactivity and impulsivity while improving focus, motivation, and memory by optimizing dopamine and norepinephrine activity in the prefrontal cortex. Extended release versions provide longer symptom relief. Potential side effects include insomnia, appetite suppression, headaches, and mood reactivity. Dosages require very gradual fine tuning based on tolerance. Take medication holidays to assess ongoing need.

Non-Stimulant Medications – Drugs like atomoxetine (Strattera), alpha-agonists such as guanfacine, and certain antidepressants target norepinephrine and serotonin instead of stimulating dopamine. They prove less potent for focus but may help those who don't tolerate stimulants well. Discuss pros and cons of each option thoroughly with your prescribing provider.

Therapy and Coaching – Ongoing counseling provides accountability, coping strategies for relationships and work, organizing tools, emotional regulation skills, and support. Cognitive behavioral therapy often proves most effective, although many modalities offer benefit. Finding the right therapist fit and specializing in ADHD takes trial and error. Consider both individual and couples counseling.

Brain Training – Working with a specialist on mindfulness practices, breathing exercises, cognitive drills, and executive functioning skills can help retrain neural pathways over time. Physical exercise also builds focus and self-discipline gradually through brain changes over months. Be patient awaiting results.

Organization Systems – External compensatory strategies help circumvent ADHD impairments in time management, planning, and memory. Wall calendars, electronic or paper planners, color coding, label makers, checklists, automatic payment systems, smart home devices, and more all provide scaffolding. Observe which methods click best for your partner.

Healthy Routines – Regular sleep, nutritious anti-inflammatory diet, physical activity, social connection, and self-care practices reduce ADHD severity. Assist in forming habits not requiring continual motivation. Swimming, yoga, light weights, time outdoors etc. boost mental clarity. Track symptoms vigilantly if diet changes.

Limiting Alcohol and Recreational Drugs – While some self-medicate ADHD with marijuana, alcohol or stimulants, these substances exacerbate challenges long-term. Strictly avoid during workdays. Support healthy outlets like relationships, hobbies, therapy and prescribed medications instead of risky self-management.

Education and Advocacy – Finally, learning everything possible about ADHD strengthens self-advocacy skills, self-acceptance, and ability to educate loved ones. Insight into ADHD as an alternative neurotype bred unique gifts and blindspots reduces stigma. Confidently seek accommodations as needed.

Treatment plans are highly personalized. Make medication and lifestyle decisions aligned with your shared values and goals. Patience, teamwork, and open communication with providers allows finding the optimal fit over time.

Holistic Approaches for Supporting Overall Wellbeing

While prescription treatments play an integral role managing diagnoses like PCOS and ADHD, holistic supportive therapies nurture total mind-body health. Incorporating certain complementary approaches enhances progress:

Nutritional Therapy – Meeting with a dietitian knowledgeable in both conditions helps tailor eating plans balancing hormones, focus, energy levels, and medical needs without extremes. Diet alone cannot cure PCOS or ADHD but optimizing nutrition bolsters progress.

Acupuncture – This traditional Chinese medicine modality uses hair-thin needles stimulating specific meridian points to reduce pain, regulate menstrual cycles, improve sleep, decrease inflammation, and treat accompanying mood disorders. It proves a helpful adjunctive therapy.

Chiropractic Care – Gentle spinal adjustments realign the nervous system, boost circulation, ease muscle tension, and reduce pain caused by postural issues or chronic stress. Integrative chiropractors offer broader nutritional and lifestyle guidance as well.

Supplements and Herbs – After checking for medication interactions, supplements like omega-3s, B complex, vitamin D, calcium, magnesium, green tea extract, and targeted herbs can support energy, cognition, and metabolic regulation. Work with an educated integrative provider on formulations and dosing.

Essential Oils – Scents like lavender, chamomile, rose, frankincense, and lemon oil help reduce anxiety, improve sleep quality, increase alertness, and manage pain through aromatherapy. Topical, inhaled, or diluted in baths, oils enhance wellness routines.

Guided Imagery and Hypnosis – These mind-body relaxation techniques foster calm and focus helping manage stress, anxiety, depression, insomnia and pain. Some providers even integrate hypnosis for building motivation around nutrition and fitness. Apps offer guided sessions too.

Biofeedback and Neurofeedback – Using sensors and computer software, these innovative interventions provide real-time feedback about physiological stress responses and brainwave patterns. In turn, clients learn to consciously regulate anxiety, pain, focus, and sleep. Sessions train long-lasting skills.

Nature and Art Therapies – Spending reflective time outdoors, hiking, or gardening combines the mental health benefits of fresh air, sunshine, stress relief, and mindfulness. Expressive artistic outlets like music, painting, dance, photography also help channel creativity and emotions.

Light Therapy – Exposure to special full spectrum light boxes mimicking natural sunlight boosts circadian rhythms, mood, alertness, and focus especially helpful in seasons with less sun. Just 10-30 minutes daily prevents SAD symptoms.

By incorporating various holistic modalities alongside standard treatments, you harness the power of integrative care in enhancing whole person wellbeing. Support your partner in finding practitioners capable of blending both perspectives.

Navigating the Emotional and Relational Impacts of Diagnoses

Receiving a diagnosis like PCOS or ADHD as an adult inevitably stirs up complex feelings from mourning lost time to relief at finally having answers. Partners play a vital role providing space for emotional processing along the journey.

Following diagnosis, use open-ended questions to explore your partner's experience:

- How are you feeling about receiving this ADHD diagnosis? Nervous, hopeful, overwhelmed?

- What old struggles and experiences are making more sense now, knowing you've had undiagnosed PCOS since puberty?

- What are the hardest parts for you about coming to terms with this diagnosis? What fears or losses arise?

- In contrast, what opportunities feel possible now with an accurate diagnosis and treatment plan?

Listen without judgment or trying to "fix" feelings. Validate the full spectrum of emotions. Share resources about others' journeys to help normalize reactions.

Next, discuss how your relationship dynamic may evolve with treatment. While immensely helpful, medications like stimulants for ADHD require adjustments. Have open conversations around changes like:

- Newfound ability to focus on conversations without constant distraction

- Improved listening and emotion regulation skills

- Better organization with household responsibilities

- More calm and less impulsive reactions

Some differences may feel jarring after years of certain patterns. Recalibrate communication styles and expectations with grace. Ultimately, the enhanced self-regulation and motivation build deeper intimacy even if it takes time to adjust.

Finally, ponder opportunities for the diagnosis to inform career paths, hobbies, living situations and approaches to parenting if applicable. Rather than something "wrong", reframing the diagnosis as a guide for thriving elicits empowerment. Define yourselves by possibilities, not limitations. With shared understanding, compassion, patience and support, embrace this roadmap to living fully in your purpose.

Forming Healthcare Teams for Integrated Care

Given the many facets involved in managing dual diagnoses, intentionally forming a diverse healthcare team provides huge advantage. Below are key practitioners to assemble for comprehensive coordinated care:

- Primary Care Doctor – This main hub coordinates referrals, interprets test results, and manages prescriptions with big picture perspective about overall health status. Ensure choosing an empathetic doctor interested in holistic care.

- PCOS Specialist – Sometimes a reproductive endocrinologist who deeply understands the nuances of hormone testing, metabolic markers, fertility impacts, latest treatment options, and multi-systemic nature.

- ADHD Psychiatrist – Psychiatrists have specialized expertise fine-tuning ADHD medications and other prescriptions to target symptoms while minimizing side effects and monitoring cardiac health.

- Therapist/Counselor – Choose a therapist well-versed in ADHD and trauma-informed modalities such as CBT, DBT, and mindfulness practices. Even if your partner feels functional, therapy provides immense stress relief and skill building.

- Registered Dietitian – Nutrition professionals guide any dietary changes, address nutritional deficiencies, ensure adequate nourishment during weight loss, and tailor meal plans to your preferences and health conditions. Beware excessive food rules.

- Functional Medicine Provider – These practitioners specialize in holistic protocols integrating targeted supplements and lifestyle medicine with standard care. Seek ones using evidence-based precision testing.

- Health Coach – Coaches help with motivation, accountability, organization systems, and consistent self-care habits. They empower sustainable lifestyle changes through supportive check-ins.

With this collaborative team actively communicating, your care feels coordinated as a whole versus fragmented. Lean on the experts respective to each aspect of treatment. Over time, fine tune your support system as needs evolve. By surrounding yourselves with wisdom and compassion, you ensure the journey never feels solitary.

Partnering in Medical Decision Making

Since PCOS and ADHD have both medical and emotional components, including your partner closely in health decisions respects their agency while benefiting the relationship. However, the right balance must be struck between abdicating all control versus dictating authoritarian demands.

Have proactive dialogues about your respective preferences and values regarding treatment plans. For example, if your partner participates in a more alternative health culture, discuss how to blend both conventional and complementary modalities for optimal balance. Or share any concerns about specific medications to find alternatives supporting both your comfort levels.

During appointments, speak up with the doctors kindly and assertively to understand all options while ensuring your partner's voice is also heard. Offer to jot down notes she may miss or forget. Help formulate questions ahead of time.

Also recognize that as her diagnoses do not directly impact your health, try to offer input as suggestions, not rigid mandates. Ultimately it must remain her choice navigating available treatments in alignment with her goals and values while taking your perspective into account.

Outside appointments, provide tangible support executing agreed upon plans – reminders about new supplements, cooking meals accommodating updated diet needs, researching potential specialist referrals. Checking in around what makes treatment feel most manageable for your particular lifestyles and priorities prevents assuming "one size fits all."

Above all, keep the communication compassionate. If you grow frustrated around follow through, reflect on what barriers her executive functioning challenges may pose rather than scolding willpower. Help brainstorm systems that set you both up for success. With team spirit, you become active collaborators, not adversaries in care.

Supporting Medication Changes and Lapses

Finding optimal ADHD medication types and dosages requires an ongoing process of careful titration and tracking responsiveness. Prepare for a marathon, not a sprint. Be especially attentive during med adjustments.

Note improvements as well as side effects together. Keep an open dialogue about benefits versus intolerable tradeoffs and communicate frequently with the prescriber until dosage feels therapeutic. Prevent harsh come downs by proactively planning refill dates and weaning down responsibly if discontinuing.

Understand that forgetting to take pills sometimes occurs given executive functioning challenges. Skip shaming about "noncompliance" which feeds unhelpful mental scripts around failure. Instead offer pragmatic help like setting phone alarms, weekly pill organizers, timers, or text reminders when away from home.

If your partner misses doses for multiple days consecutively or takes arbitrary medication holidays, do express concern compassionately. Explore any barriers like side effect frustrations, denial around diagnosis, or ambivalence derailing consistency. Remind her you just want to see her feeling their best. But refrain from policing tone.

ADHD medication changes require teamwork and tremendous courage facing uncertainties. Your unwavering support through the process speaks louder than any nagging. Offer dependability when her brain struggles with follow through. And through each transition, let your care speak louder than her symptoms.

Seeking Counseling and Community Support

Finally, don't underestimate the power of counseling and community for promoting understanding around your partner's diagnoses. While medicines treat acute symptoms, mental health interventions and peer support address shame, relationships, and long-held negative beliefs undermining thriving.

A therapist offering cognitive behavioral therapy, mindfulness training, and compassion practices helps develop essential coping skills, attachment security, and emotional regulation - keys for maximizing medical treatments. If couples counseling fits your budget, even occasional sessions improve dynamic insights.

Peer support groups – in person or online - provide the immensely healing medicine of shared experiences combating isolation. Connecting "offline" with those traveling similar roads delivers hope, wisdom and belonging. Excellent options range from ADHD meetups to PCOS forums and conferences.

Of course, your most vital support will remain the unconditional understanding and kindness you offer day-to-day. But by surrounding yourselves with compassionate professionals and communities, you gain further tools and wisdom for the path ahead. With doubled hands and hearts, step forward together toward deeper healing.

Staying Organized: Tips for Managing Daily Life and Tasks

When your partner lives with dual diagnoses like PCOS and ADHD, organization rarely comes naturally. Chronic disarray often pervades their physical and mental spaces adding frustration to daily functioning. As an understanding partner, you can implement strategies mitigating the chaos with patience and compassion.

Rather than criticism, provide realistic structured solutions collaboratively. Help fill gaps that executive functioning challenges create without disempowering agency. With creativity and teamwork, build bridges between intention and action. Let's explore tips promoting focus, order, and flow amidst the whirlwind.

Establishing Daily Routines

At the foundation of organization lies consistent routines. Without anchored structure, each day feels adrift. Routines create rhythms instilling a sense of control when hormones, distraction, and impulse continually disrupt.

Start by identifying your partner's peak productivity window so key tasks align with optimal energy. Also capture preferred sleep and wake times accounting for ADHD delayed sleep phase.

Build routines around these chronobiology realities, not the shoulds of conventional time norms which set your partner up for failure. Protect their biological needs.

Next layer in essential self-care like nutrition, activity, quiet time, and social connection at appropriate intervals. scattered ADD tendencies thrive on rituals. Penciling in these priorities first prevents neglecting them when demands compete.

Finally, plug in other fixed obligations around this scaffolding – shift times, recurring meetings, medical appointments, etc. Maintaining open blocks for flexibility remains important, however. Rigidity backfires.

Post the schedule prominently. Review it together weekly making any adaptations needed. Consistency and accountability help routines stick long-term versus abandoned in overwhelm. Gradually the patterns feel steadying, not suffocating.

Mastering Morning and Evening Routines

Mornings and evenings represent crucial times where consistent routines minimize later chaos. Bookend days with centering, productivity, and self-care.

AM Jumpstarts

- Hydrate immediately upon waking with a full glass of water. Dehydration derails cognition.

- Open blinds first thing to trigger melatonin shutoff and circadian rhythm alignment.

- Exercise or meditate before digital stimulation. These neurochemical boosts power focus.

- Eat a protein-rich breakfast. Complex carbs alone lead to mid-morning crashes.

- Take medications/supplements immediately with food. Don't lapse before leaving home.

- Check calendar and set daily intentions. Making a plan beats reacting.

- Gather belongings needed for the day by the door. Prevent frantic last minute scrambling.

PM Wind Downs

- Use the commute home to unwind with preferred music or a podcast.

- Change into comfy clothes and set aside work materials. Home is for rest.

- Schedule evening priorities like family time, making food, and extra work. Don't get derailed vegging out.

- Note tomorrow's agenda. Prep bags/supplies needed for morning efficiency.

- Have an evening relaxation ritual like reading, stretching, or crafting.

- Power down electronics 30-60 minutes before bed. Blue light delays sleep.

- Spend time cuddling or connecting with your partner before sleep.

- Keep nightstand free of clutter for serene sleep space.

Structure bookending days prevents the chaos avalanche so common with executive function challenges. Follow routines even when unmotivated. Consistency builds the grooves.

Weekly Planning and Prep

While daily routines establish regularity, your partner also needs systems ensuring broader organization. Dedicate time each week to big picture planning and preparation empowering productivity and lowering stress.

Sunday Planning

- Review upcoming week's appointments and obligations in a planner. Note periods reserved for focusing on big projects.

- Create a running task list with checkboxes to satisfy accomplishment endorphins.

- Schedule self-care activities ensuring they claim space on the calendar.

- Meal plan dinners and prep recipes in advance when possible. Stock up on grab and go breakfasts/lunches.

- Straighten, declutter, and clean to reset home environment reducing overwhelm.

- Mentally prepare for the week by listing hopes, gratitudes, and priorities.

Ongoing Sunday Prep

- Sort mail, file bills to pay, schedule time for administrative tasks.

- Review calendar and planner side-by-side to identify any gaps or conflicts needing adjustment.

- Catch up on meal prep if needed for healthy grab and go breakfasts and lunches.

- Refill medication boxes. Add recurring prescription refills to digital calendar.

- Make shopping list noting must-have grocery staples and household needs.

- Check work bag contents, gas tank fill level, and charge devices.

Planning ahead each week reduces the mental clutter trying to recall obligations last minute. Preparation breeds confidence entering the work week aligned with purpose rather than scrambling.

Harnessing Bullet Journals

For ADHD minds, digital calendars and long format planning feel overwhelming. Bullet journals streamline organization through succinct rapid logging in dedicated notebooks. The creativity and flexibility proves more palatable than rigid apps.

Help your partner design a bullet journal system honoring their quirks. It can incorporate any components fitting their needs:

- Running rapid log of tasks and events as they arise

- Monthly and future log for major appointments, trips etc

- Habit tracking for consistency like medications, fitness, nutrition

- Brain dumps to empty mental clutter onto paper

- Calming artistic touches and washi tape for fun

- Streaming consciousness creative writing or poetry

- Visual mood boards from magazine cutouts

- Gratitude logging and affirmations

The beauty of bullet journaling lies in the ability to customize it intuitively in ways technology can't replicate. Let your partner add or modify elements at will. When executive functioning bogs them down, opening the journal provides clarity.

Optimizing Digital Tools and Devices

While analog systems help many partners with ADHD, digital organization platforms and devices offer benefits too. Tech creates accountability, reminders, and ease managing life admin when used strategically.

Streamline with Apps – Consolidate calendars, checklists, documents and projects into integratable platforms like Google Suite or Microsoft Office. Link email, calendar, and drive for seamless access.

Automate Finances – Online banking with auto-pay, recurring transfers, and budget tracker apps rein in impulse spending and prevents missed payments. Get paperless statements.

Voice Assist – Smart speakers to play reminders, lists, and music hands-free help multitask. They integrate home devices too.

Text Reminders – Use free services like Remind101 for sending scheduled medication, appointment, and task alerts. Customize frequency.

Digital Bulletin Board – Use Pinterest or photo albums to compile visual references in one place – wish lists, recipe ideas, travel goals etc.

Real-Time Shared Lists – Mobile apps like Cozi give family members synchronized grocery lists, to do's, and calendars. Great for coordinating schedules.

Focus Devices – Noise cancelling headphones, apps that limit distracting websites, and digital white noise machines reduce mental clutter.

Tech can overwhelm so avoid adopting too many new tools at once. Note which digital systems feel intuitive and streamlining versus added hassle. Curate your toolkit.

Getting Paperwork and Files Organized

Paper piles breed anxiety yet organizing documents often feels daunting. Make it more manageable by tackling one area at a time. Maintain systems in digestible increments.

Stash Nearby Supplies – Keep frequently used filing supplies easily accessible - stapler, paper clips, tape, pens, extra folders etc. Eliminate hunts when motivation strikes.

Sort and Purge – Spend 15 minutes sorting papers into "action needed", "file", and "toss" piles. Process actions immediately before paperwork again piles up.

Calendar Admin Time – Schedule 30-60 minutes weekly for filing papers, paying bills, scheduling appointments and other clerical tasks. Protecting focus time prevents avoidance.

One Note In/Out Boxes– Centralized trays for incoming and outgoing items helps quickly triage and route docs.

Digital Scan – Apps like Scanner Pro allow quick digitization of important documents into cloud storage. Organize scans like digital files. Reduces paper overload.

Label Everything – Use color coded folders, sticky tabs, and handwritten notes labeling storage boxes/binders by topic for intuitive filing. Create a key.

Minimize Clutter – Avoid stacks on desks and exposed shelving which contribute to visual chaos. Contain clutter in drawers, bins and baskets out of sight.

Room by room, conquer paper disorder and establish systems preventing future avalanches. Maintaining neat workflows allows documents to file themselves naturally.

Optimizing Handbag, Work Bag, and Wallet

Few things disrupt a day like frantically emptying bags searching for lost keys, wallets or phones. These prime ADHD trap zones require strategic organization.

Designate Basics – Certain essentials like ID, insurance cards, debit/credit card, cash, lip balm and charger always remain in wallet. Use minimalist wallets with designated compartments.

Keys on Lanyard – Attach keys to a badge lanyard with ID. Wear lanyard during purse use so keys stay visible. Carabiner clips also secure.

Take Inventory – Use a small notebook or planner to jot down each item as its placed in purse or work bag. Review inventory before leaving places.

Slim Down Extras – Limit unnecessary items carried. Set reminders transferring bulky work documents back to their office storage spots.

Utilize Pockets – Use zippered compartments or inner pouches to separately contain items prone to sinking to the bottom like headphones or lip gloss.

Take Photos – Snap a picture of the bag fully packed and organized. Refer to it when feeling the urge to needlessly dump everything out.

Clean It Out – Make a weekly ritual of removing clutter, cleaning linings, and wiping down electronics and water bottles stored in bags.

Checklists prevent losing track of belongings within those black hole bags we carry everywhere. Frequently used items deserve designated homes. Keeping bags light also minimizes mess.

With compassion and collaboration, organization evolves from burden to bonding experience. Don't expect perfection. Progress comes gradually through trying systems, troubleshooting what falls through cracks, and pivoting strategies over time.

Trust organization is a process, not a personality trait. Your partner's desire for order remains strong even if their executive functioning fails them. Support their intentions with understanding.

Remember, routines deeply anchor those who feel adrift in the rapids of distraction. Order alleviates self-judgement about perceived shortcomings. And pragmatic solutions prevent frustration from hijacking your connection.

While each day presents challenges, recognize your partner's strengths too – creativity, passion, loyalty, resourcefulness. Build environments nurturing those superpowers as well. With your steady partnership calming the storms, clarity emerges one step at a time.

Emotional Support: Being the Pillar Without Being Overwhelmed

Partners of those managing chronic health conditions often naturally fall into the role of steadfast emotional pillar holding the relationship strong when times get tough. However, absorbing the perpetual storms of distress your loved one faces risks depleting your own reserves over time, leading to resentment. How do you balance bearing their burdens with setting boundaries around emotional capacity? Let's explore strategies for providing support, cultivating self-care, and getting help when needed. Your empathy must come from a well of energy that you actively replenish.

Validating their Emotional Experiences

The first step lies in truly accepting the spectrum of emotions your partner expresses stemming from their dual diagnoses – including the dark, messy ones like anger, hopelessness, or grief. Avoid trying to immediately "fix" painful feelings. Just be present.

Rather than defending or explaining away their symptoms when emotions run high, pause to listen and understand. Ask what thoughts underlie the feelings to deepen insight about their inner world.

Reflect back what you hear without judgment and with empathy:

"I know how upsetting and discouraging managing these symptoms must feel each day."

"This anger is coming from a place of pain about the effects you didn't ask for."

"You have every right to mourn the way this condition has disrupted the joys you imagined for life."

"I can't fully grasp what it's like in your shoes, but I appreciate you helping me understand."

Let them fully express their authentic feelings. Emotional acceptance provides the safety for hope to ultimately emerge amid the darkness. Suppressing their challenges for sake of positivity only breeds distance.

Offer tangible help navigating the emotions. Suggest healthy outlets like journaling, support groups, counseling or complementary therapies to aid processing. Help schedule these self-care respites which replenish their inner well.

When they're caught in storms of lament and self-criticism, gently redirect to recall previous examples of resilience or wins. Help counterbalance discouraging narratives with hope.

Finding Calm in Chaos Together

In the eye of distress and uncertainty their diagnoses trigger, your peaceful presence steadies. Help cultivate daily anchors of calm and meaning amidst the chaos which throws equilibrium off.

Schedule quality time together pursuing activities that build connection and lift spirits - making meals, being in nature, enjoying shared hobbies, volunteering for causes you care about.

Practice stress-relieving rituals as a couple like meditating, massaging one another or soaking in epsom baths. Don't underestimate simple pleasures.

Keep a gratitude list of all blessings big and small. Reciting these gifts and accomplishments when darkness looms restores perspective.

Remind them their value is never defined by productive output. Help release the pressure to handle everything flawlessly. Progress over perfection matters most.

Work together to reduce sources of negative stress and activity overload. Evaluate if obligations deplete more than uplift. What demands can be dropped or delegated?

When they apologize for needing extensive support, reply "I'm always here to help shoulder the rough patches. We support each other no matter what."

Reframe setbacks as opportunities to problem solve together versus reasons to berate themselves. Maintain a spirit of "us versus the issue, not each other."

Your unwavering belief in their abilities to overcome and thrive carries them through stormy seas, back to sanctuary. Hold fast to hope.

Setting Healthy Boundaries Around Your Limits

Being an unconditional emotional pillar for your partner does require boundaries so you don't sacrifice your own needs and wellbeing. Burnout prevents truly being present. Know your capacity and communicate limits sensitively.

If constantly hearing solely negatives starts weighing you down, gently redirect the conversation:

"I want to be your safe space to vent so you don't hold this all in. At the same time, staying stuck in problem focus amplifies despair. Could we balance discussions about some of the hopeful aspects too?"

"My spirit feels drained today. Can we connect by cooking together or watching a comedy instead of processing more worries right now?"

When requests for support become unrealistic, offer compromise:

"I wish I could join every doctor appointment to take notes, but my work schedule makes that really tough. What if we recorded visits on our phones so I can be involved from home?"

"I know how frustrating parenting is some days with the ADHD challenges. I'm happy to take over mornings before work. But let's plan who handles which times to avoid me burning out."

If criticisms about your support approach feel overly harsh, express your feelings while reaffirming commitment:

"I feel hurt when my efforts to help are met with criticism or irritation. But I'm still here. Let's talk through better ways I can show up."

"When every solution I suggest gets rejected, I start taking it really personally. Can you help me understand what doesn't feel supportive so I can modify my approach?"

"I know you lash out at me when you're in pain. But I ask that you find ways to vent anger that don't attack my character."

You can lovingly safeguard your emotional needs while remaining engaged. Measure out compassion in sustainable chunks. Your partner will benefit most from a present peaceful you, not a depleted shell.

Helping vs Enabling

It's natural to want to intervene solving every struggle your partner faces. But in your eagerness to assuage their troubles, take care not to inadvertently enable unhelpful behaviors or thinking patterns. The healthiest support empowers their autonomy.

For example, completing tasks on their behalf when frustration mounts often provides short-term relief but deprives them of opportunities to build skills managing ADHD symptoms independently. It's a slippery slope between helping and enabling dependency.

Similarly, rushing to soothe every worry and self-criticism stops them from learning tools to self-regulate emotions and inner negative chatter. Don't immediately solve problems they're fully capable of handling themselves.

You walk the line between being loving assistant and possessive enabler. Have patience letting your partner struggle productively through challenges building their own coping muscles and earned confidence.

The most empowering support scaffolds just enough – helping them devise systems for self-organization, gently nudging them to start difficult conversations themselves, role modeling healthy thinking patterns through your lived example.

Master the art of holding back unsolicited advice while still providing safety nets. Offer support that props them up rather than holds them back. Help your partner learn to fly solo even if the process feels bumpy. The falls make the flying sweeter.

Relinquishing Control Over Their Treatment Journey

One of the greatest acts of love is letting your partner steer their own health journey. Avoid playing authoritarian doctor. While your input adds helpful perspective, their diagnoses ultimately impact their lived experience most. Allow autonomy over managing care.

Respect their right to start and discontinue medications or specific diets on their own terms even if you fervently disagree. Different treatments affect you as the partner far less directly. Make suggestions not demands.

If new approaches seem to deteriorate their condition, kindly share your observations then let them come to their own conclusions when ready. People more fully embrace change when self-directed.

Support their treatment choices even if very different from what you would select. Their path to thriving may veer away from the conventional at times. Keep an open mind.

Let your role be an unconditional listening ear they can fully be themselves around, not a parental enforcer. They show up best for healing when self-motivated versus pressured to please you.

The most empowering partners adopt a "You lead, I support" mentality regarding this journey that isn't yours to control. Your unwavering faith in their inner wisdom provides the safety net to keep trying new roads until answers unfold.

Managing Stress Around the Unknowns

The uncertainty chronic health conditions breed often overwhelms loved ones. Fears arise not knowing if or when new symptoms may flare or progress.

Tolerating ambiguity feels excruciating. However, anticipating hypothetical worst cases wastes present moments. Manage worries through:

Mindfulness - Get out of future spiral thoughts by paying attention to right now - sights, sounds, sensations. Breathe slowly. Take in the stillness and stability surrounding temporary health storms.

Perspective - When your mind leaps to catastrophic "what ifs" about decline or debility, balance those with factual realities about the patient, stable condition your partner currently enjoys.

Counter-balance anxiety with logic.

Presence - Rather than endlessly researching obscure risks online, redirect attention to tangible actions of loving service you can focus on day-to-day like preparing nourishing meals or organizing medication refills. Active care alleviates worry.

Release - Journal stream of consciousness style allowing yourself to vent every pinned up fear and frustration to release their grip. Then burn or shred the pages. Let imagined outcomes go.

Meaning - Get involved with communities supporting your partner's condition to see the incredible hope, resilience and purpose that arises even facing challenges. Surround despair with meaning.

Your calmness anchors your partner's worries. Manage your own stressors consciously so they don't compound an already full emotional load. Breathe through fears of the unknown, so now feels peaceful.

Supporting Other Relationships Impacted

Finally, recognize your partner's diagnoses may strain broader family dynamics and friendships when misunderstandings arise or limitations feel unclear. Play a mediating role educating loved ones.

If parents, siblings or friends make thoughtless comments clearly hurtful to your partner, pull them aside privately later to provide perspective:

"Kelly doesn't resist family events to be anti-social. Crowds and noise just get really overwhelming with her sensory issues. Can we help adjust group gatherings to be more ADHD friendly for her?"

"Rob isn't shirking work responsibilities. You have to understand ADHD executive functioning and focus challenges make his job much harder. Let's have some compassion about the disability he wrestles with."

"Her mood swings don't mean she doesn't love you. PCOS hormones and pain wear on anyone. She needs support, not judgment."

Offer to share educational resources to promote empathy and problematically bridge rifts.

Remind loved ones progress is often incremental. Make space for their learning curve aligning with your partner's health journey. With gentle guidance, transform relationships into healing sources instead of added burdens.

Being the sturdy emotional anchor your partner needs doesn't require martyrdom. Set yourself up for sustainable success by honoring needs and capacity. Let others share the weight through counselors or support groups. Prioritize nourishing self-care habits that replenish your spirit.

Most importantly, release self-pressure to erase all suffering. Your role is not to fix but to listen, understand and accept the spectrum of emotions that arise. Through skillful boundaries and compassion for all, become the safe harbor in every storm. Where they feel cherished exactly as they are, healing unfolds naturally. Your steadfast light guides the way.

Meal Planning for ADHD and PCOS

Strategic meal planning and nutritious food choices can make a significant difference managing ADHD and PCOS. Let's explore tips and recipes for breakfasts, lunches, dinners and snacks optimizing focus, balancing hormones and blood sugar, improving gut health, and providing steady energy.

Crafting Balanced Breakfasts

Mornings often set the trajectory for your day. Eating a balanced breakfast with protein, fiber, and healthy fats helps stabilize blood sugar and dopamine levels boosting concentration, mood, and metabolism.

Here are nourishing ADHD and PCOS-friendly breakfast ideas:

- Veggie Egg Muffin – Lightly beat 2 eggs. Sauté chopped spinach and mushrooms. Add egg mixture to greased muffin tin. Bake 15-20 minutes at 375F. Serve with melon.

- Chia Pudding – Mix 1/4 cup chia seeds with 1 cup dairy or non-dairy milk. Refrigerate overnight. Top with berries and slivered almonds in the morning.

- Avocado Toast – Mash half an avocado onto whole grain toast. Top with Everything Bagel seasoning, smoked salmon or fried egg for non-vegan option. Serve with citrus slices.

- Overnight Oats – Combine oats, milk, yogurt, cinnamon, and nut butter. Refrigerate overnight. Top with berries.

- Tofu Scramble Tacos – Sauté extra firm tofu crumbles with onion, peppers and spinach. Wrap in corn tortillas or serve over greens.

- Tahini Banana Smoothie – Blend milk, banana, peanut butter, vanilla, and tahini. Add ice.

- Smoked Salmon and Cream Cheese Lettuce Wraps – Top Boston lettuce leaves with smoked salmon, scallions, and dill cream cheese.

Make a batch of quick bread or muffins on the weekend to grab on busier weekday mornings. Store pre-cut fruits and veggies to throw into morning smoothies too. Having balanced components ready prevents grabbing sugary convenience breakfasts when morning executive functioning feels impaired.

Nourishing ADHD and PCOS Lunches

Packing balanced lunches fosters afternoon energy, mood stability, and focus through the post-meal blood sugar slump many experience. Build lunches combining fiber, plant protein, smart carbs, and healthy fats.

Lunch suggestions:

- Mason Jar Salad – Layer chopped greens, quinoa or chickpeas, veggies, nuts, dressing in a jar. Invert onto plate at lunch.

- Loaded Vegetarian Baked Potato – Baked potato topped with chili or sautéed mushrooms, spinach, and hummus or dairy-free cheese. It would be recommended to use red potatoes.

- Burrito Bowl – Cooked quinoa, black beans, fajita veggies, salsa, guacamole, and Greek yogurt.

- Falafel Pita – Stuffed with falafel, tomatoes, cucumbers, hummus and tzatziki or vegan ranch dressing.

- Buddha Bowl – Mixed greens topped with roasted sweet potato, edamame, avocado, pepitas. Dressed with olive oil and vinegar.

- Cauliflower Rice Tabouli Salad – Finely chop cauliflower florets into rice-like pieces. Combine with tomatoes, cucumber, parsley, mint, lemon, olive oil.

- Lentil Soup – Hearty lentil and veggie soup with side salad. Sprinkle nuts or seeds for crunch.

Double recipes making extra portions for lunches throughout the week. Include fresh fruit, roasted chickpeas, veggies with hummus or guacamole, and yogurt with nuts/seeds for satisfying balanced sides. Staying fueled prevents afternoon energy crashes.

Wholesome ADHD and PCOS Dinners

After busy days, keep dinner nutrition robust but easy. Combining veggies, plant proteins and whole grains makes balancing blood sugar effortless. Get creative with seasonings, herbs, spices, and garnishes.

Simple yet nourishing dinner ideas include:

- Sheet Pan Fajitas – Arrange sliced bell peppers and onions with seasoned black beans on a sheet pan. Roast then wrap with fixings in tortillas or lettuce.

- Loaded Baked Sweet Potato – Bake sweet potato. Top with black beans, salsa, avocado and Greek yogurt.

- Pesto Pasta – Toss whole grain pasta with homemade or prepared pesto. Serve with chicken or white beans along with steamed broccoli.

- Breaded Eggplant Parmesan – Slice eggplant, coat in breadcrumbs, bake until crisp. Top with tomato sauce and dairy-free mozzarella. Serve with salad.

- Quinoa Power Bowl – Cooked quinoa topped with roasted veggies, hemp seeds, and ginger dressing.

- Chickpea Curry – Sauté onion, then simmer coconut milk and curry powder. Add spinach and chickpeas. Serve over rice with cucumber raita.

- Fish Tacos – Bake seasoned white fish. Serve in corn tortillas with cabbage slaw and avocado crema. Enjoy with corn on the cob.

Multitask meal prep while getting movement. Chop veggies while kids play or lift weights. Grill or roast extra portions to use creatively throughout the week in salads, wraps, bowls and soups - saving time. Keep weeknight dinners nourishing.

Snacking Strategically with ADHD and PCOS

Between meals, small snacks prevent energy crashes and curb impulsive unhealthy cravings those with ADHD often battle. Combine protein, fiber and healthy fat in snacks.

Smart snacking options include:

- Apple or celery slices with nut butter

- Greek yogurt mixed with chia seeds and berries

- Edamame pods

- Hardboiled egg and sliced veggies

- Leftover salmon with whole grain crackers

- Kale chips made from torn kale tossed in olive oil and baked

- Trail mix with nuts, seeds, coconut, dark chocolate

- Oatmeal energy bites made with dates, oats, nut or seed butter

- Smoothies with spinach, banana, nut butter and milk/alternative milk

- Rice cakes topped with smashed avocado and lemon pepper

- Homemade granola bars with nuts, seeds, dried fruit, oats

Prepare bins of preportioned snacks like energy bites, trail mix, sliced fruits and veggies during a quiet weekend time to grab without thought during your busiest ADHD moments. Quick balanced snacks prevent poor impulse eating.

ADHD and PCOS Gut Healthy Bowls

Nourishing the gut microbiome with fermented foods, bone broth, probiotic foods and adequate fiber stabilizes mood, focus, hormones and metabolism in both ADHD and PCOS. Try incorporating these gut health boosters:

Pickled Food Bowls – Combine pickled ginger, sauerkraut, and kimchi with rice and protein. The tangy flavors and probiotic boost aid digestion.

Miso Soup with Seaweed – Make broth with bone broth powder, diced tofu, miso paste, seaweed and mushrooms for an mineral rich probiotic soup.

Overnight Oats with Yogurt – Soak steel cut oats in yogurt and almond milk overnight. Top with fruit the next morning for prebiotic fiber to feed probiotics.

Kombucha Smoothies – Add a splash of kombucha juice to smoothies instead of sugary juice for a fermented tang. Use ginger or berries to mask sharpness.

Bone Broth Noodle Soup – Use bone broth as the base for chicken noodle soup or Pho with rice noodles. Sip the mineral rich broth.

Green Smoothie with Sauerkraut Juice – Blend your green smoothie then stir in a tablespoon of sauerkraut juice for the probiotic boost. The fruit masks the taste.

Feeding beneficial gut flora helps modulate systemic inflammation contributing to ADHD, PCOS, and mood issues. Work gut nourishment into meals.

Anti-Inflammatory Foods and Spices

Chronic inflammation worsens many ADHD and PCOS symptoms. Cooling internal fire through anti-inflammatory nutrition aids overall function and feelings of well being.

Incorporate more:

- Omega-3s rich foods - Salmon, sardines, walnuts, flax, chia

- Leafy greens - Spinach, kale, lettuces, chard

- Colorful veggies - Broccoli, tomatoes, carrots, squash

- Herbs - Turmeric, cinnamon, rosemary, thyme

- Tea - Green tea, white tea, hibiscus tea

- Dark chocolate - Opt for at least 70% cocoa content

- Fruit - Berries, oranges, pineapple, apples, cherries

- Beans and lentils - Kidney, garbanzo, black beans, peas

- Mushrooms - Cremini, maitake, shiitake

- Hemp and pumpkin seeds provide anti-inflammatory minerals

- Tart cherry juice has compounds reducing inflammation

Spices like ginger, cayenne, garlic, and turmeric add anti-inflammatory oomph
to dishes easily. An anti-inflammatory diet eases systemic irritation aggravating
ADHD and PCOS symptoms long-term. Be patient watching inflammation
subside through nutrition over time.

Nourishing the ADHD Brain

Certain nutrients play key supportive roles fueling ADHD brains by improving
dopamine transmission, protecting neurons, and reducing inflammation.

Emphasize foods and spices providing:

- Protein - Fish, poultry, tofu, eggs, dairy, legumes, nuts

- Omega-3s - Salmon, flax, walnuts, chia

- Antioxidants - Berries, citrus fruits, leafy greens, green tea

- Zinc - Seafood, spinach, nuts and seeds

- B Vitamins - Salmon, eggs, whole grains, leafy greens

- Magnesium - Spinach, pumpkin seeds, almonds, black beans

- Iron - Spinach, grass-fed beef, lentils, pumpkin seeds

- Vitamin D - Fatty fish, eggs, fortified dairy alternatives

- Probiotics - Yogurt, kefir, kimchi, miso, kombucha

An overall balanced diet with focus on the nutrients above builds cognitive resilience managing ADHD. Protecting brain health through food pays exponential dividends long-term.

Hormone Balancing Meals for PCOS

Certain dietary approaches help regulate insulin, inflammation, cortisol and sex hormones minimizing PCOS symptoms:

Lower Glycemic - Emphasize foods like nuts, seeds, legumes, whole grains and vegetables that digest slower to balance blood sugar. Sweet potatoes and quinoa, for example, are better options than white potatoes or white rice.

Increase Fiber - Aim for 25-35 grams of fiber daily from vegetables, fruits, whole grains, nuts and seeds to support the liver and stabilize insulin.

Healthy Fats - Incorporate more anti-inflammatory fats like olive oil, avocados, salmon, walnuts. They balance hormones and provide key nutrients.

Adaptogen Foods - Incorporate ashwagandha, maca and ginseng which help modulate cortisol and stress supporting hormonal wellbeing.

Detoxifying - Eat more cruciferous veggies, berries, garlic, lemon, flax and greens that assist liver detoxification and estrogen clearance.

While no specific diet cures PCOS, thoughtful meal planning helps alleviate systemic strain and hormone symptoms. Developing balanced yet enjoyable eating habits supports long-term hormone health.

ADHD and PCOS Blood Sugar Friendly Desserts

You needn't avoid all sweets in the name of health. The key is balancing indulgences with nutritious meals. Select treats made with some protein, fiber and healthy fats to prevent blood sugar spikes and crashes.

Some smarter dessert options include:

- Greek yogurt berry parfaits topped with nuts and dark chocolate

- Apples baked with cinnamon, nutmeg, raisins and a crust made of oats

- Chocolate peanut butter energy bites made with dates, nut butter, cocoa powder, rolled oats

- Frozen banana "ice cream" blended up with nut butter, cocoa powder and a splash of milk

- Chia seed chocolate pudding made with cacao powder, chia seeds, milk of choice and sweetened to taste with maple syrup or pitted dates

- Dark chocolate avocado mousse made with avocado, cocoa powder, vanilla, and sweetener

- Baked pumpkin spice doughnuts with almond flour, pumpkin puree, eggs, cinnamon and nutmeg

- Single serving skillet cookie with oats, nut butter, vanilla, and mix-ins like chocolate chips then baked

When cravings strike, you have healthier options curbing the urge without totally depriving yourself or spiking glucose. Savory balanced snacks also help tame sweets cravings before reaching for candy or ice cream.

ADHD and PCOS Meal Prep Strategies

Streamline nourishing meal planning by embracing a few meal prep strategies:

- Double recipes making extras to freeze for grab and go lunches or dinners later in the week

- Roast sheet pans of vegetables on Sunday to add as easy sides to meals all week

- Cook a big batch of whole grains like quinoa or brown rice on weekends for quick weekday additions

- Wash and chop vegetables and fruits soon as you get home from the grocery store

- Stock your freezer with healthier convenience items like premade smoothies and individual portioned soups, stews, and chilis

- Make a big egg or oatmeal bake on weekends that provides protein-packed breakfasts you just reheat

- Have ingredients for easy meals like tacos, salads, and sheet pan baked salmon ready to combine with little thought

When executive functioning feels compromised, you reduce decision fatigue having components ready to throw together balanced meals easily. Embrace support strategies.

ADHD Kitchen Organization Tips

Creating an efficient, organized kitchen setup minimizes overwhelm preparing food with ADHD:

- Label bins/baskets clearly for pantry items, equipment and food categories like snacks or baking goods. Labels help everything find intuitive homes.

- Store items used most regularly on countertops or eye-level shelving for easy access without rummaging like spices, oils, condiments and cooking tools.

- Use clear storage containers so contents are visible without opening. Lazy susans also keep items accessible.

- Arrange cooking zones by task - food prep, oven, stovetop, sink/cleanup. Keep necessities for each task in that area.

- Minimize clutter with hooks, racks, pegboards and shelving to give everything a designated space off surfaces.

- Post helpful lists like weeknight meal ideas, pantry staples to restock, knife uses, and measurement conversions somewhere easily visible.

While systems benefit everyone, those with ADHD particularly thrive with structured orderly environments reducing stimulus and decision overload in the kitchen.

Nourishing the Body and Spirit

An overall balanced diet fuels both optimal physical and mental health managing ADHD and PCOS. Equally important, foster positive relationships with food and your body. Make meals a calm enjoyable oasis through the chaos of chronic conditions. Prioritize the pleasures - flavors, aromas, textures, colors and memories food evokes. Let each dish nourish your whole spirit.

Daily Routines: Creating Structure for Better Mental Health

When your partner lives with conditions like PCOS and ADHD, consistency rarely comes easily. The executive functioning deficits and hormonal fluctuations intrinsic to these diagnoses can make steady routines feel impossible to maintain. However, personalizing predictability provides a vital anchor stabilizing the storms.

Routines reduce decision fatigue, instill a needed sense of control, improve self-esteem as tasks get accomplished, and make self-care a default habit. Structure breeds mental wellness. Together you can creatively build in routines balancing flexibility with function. Let's explore strategies for morning, evening, and lifestyle rituals enhancing mental health through each day's rhythms.

Morning Routines To Start Days Grounded

Mornings often set the trajectory for the whole day. A relaxing, intentional morning routine generates a sense of groundedness and order, while a frenetic, unstructured start fuels overwhelm. Help your partner begin each morning with routines instilling calm and purpose.

Wake Mindfully – Avoid jarring alarms. Use lamps, music or sunrise clocks to gently transition wakefulness. Savor a few moments of soft breathing and gratitude before rising.

Hydrate Immediately – Drink water immediately upon standing to rehydrate and kickstart digestion and circulation. Dehydration contributes to brain fog.

Move Every Morning – Get circulation going with yoga, stretching, or brief cardio. This energizes, balances hormones, and stimulates cognition.

Eat a Nutritious Breakfast – Don't skip breakfast - nutrients fuel focus and stable blood sugar. Include fiber, protein and anti-inflammatory fats.

Practice Affirmations – While sipping coffee or tea, reflect on uplifting mantras like "I am at peace", "I have everything I need inside me now" or "Today I will channel my gifts."

Set Daily Intentions – Each morning, define 1-3 specific intentions to anchor the day's purpose and priorities. Writing these down provides clarity.

Get Ready Slowly – Avoid mad dashes. Play preferred music and savor some quiet alone time dressing, grooming and preparing for the day mindfully.

Review the Schedule – Before commuting, check calendar and make note of any appointments, tasks or events coming up. Mentally prepare.

Ritualizing the precious morning hours breeds stability from the inside out. When the first moments of each day feel grounded, it powerfully ripples through everything that follows.

Soothing Evening Rituals For Restorative Sleep

Just as mornings establish the stage for the many hours ahead, bedtime routines help clear residual stress and activate the body's relaxation response for restful sleep. Help your partner build rituals supporting unwinding.

Unplug – Limit stimulating blue light exposure from TV, phones and computers ideally for 1-2 hours before bed. Read or have disconnected conversations instead.

Take a Warm Bath – Baths two hours before bed cue the brain to release sleep hormones like melatonin. Add epsom or essential oils.

Sip Calming Tea – Chamomile, passionflower, lemon balm and cinnamon teas boost sleep quality.

Stretch – Light yoga poses release muscle tension accumulated from the day's activities promoting comfort.

Write Worries Down – Journaling or making a bulleted brain dump list clears anxious thoughts so they don't keep one awake.

Use Essential Oils – Lavender, bergamot, clary sage, and marjoram used in baths, diffusers or topically aid relaxation.

Read Paper Books – Reading physical books versus scrolling easy-to-absorb content allows the brain to wind down naturally.

Enjoy Affection – Hug, kiss, and cuddle your partner reminding one another of your care. Sweet words prevent drifting off on a disconnected note.

Keep It Cool – Ensure the bedroom is comfortably cool. Hot temperatures disrupt melatonin release and prevent deep restorative sleep.

Make evenings an oasis from the stimulation and worries of the day. When nights transition gradually into serenity, sleep comes more easily. The routines you support become their lifeline.

Weekly Planning Rituals For Organization

While daily routines breed stability, your partner also benefits from weekly planning rituals to instill proactive organization. Scheduling these administrative tasks ensures they actually happen amidst busy weeks.

Choose a consistent time each week to:

Review the Master Calendar – Sit together and review all appointments, deadlines, and commitments coming up for the next 1-2 weeks. Add any missing items and make adjustments as needed.

Make a To-Do List – Compile a thorough list of any tasks needing completion this week such as calling doctors, errands, chores, paperwork and upcoming projects. List them by priority.

Assign Responsibilities – Decide who will handle each to do, household duty, or appointment. Divide and conquer what's reasonable.

Meal Plan – Brainstorm healthy dinner ideas and grocery list needs. Prep recipes in advance when possible. Stock up on grab and go snacks/meals.

Schedule Self-Care – Plug in time for mindfulness practices, hobbies, dates, long baths, etc. Treat self-nourishment as any other obligation.

Review Finances – Reconcile any spending from the week. Set financial goals and budget categories if needed. Automate bills to limit late fees.

Order Supplements – Ensure any supplements, vitamins, or medications needing refills are reordered with delivery before running out. Set text or app refill reminders.

File Paperwork – Process any pending documents like mail, forms, bills. Don't let documents pile up into avalanches.

Straighten Up – Declutter surfaces and key zones like the entryway, office, kitchen counters. An orderly environment clears mental space.

Ritualizing regular upkeep spotlights potential issues before small stresses compound. Protect weekly administrator time together to synchronize life. Consistent planning prevents chaos.

Bedrock Daily Self-Care Habits

Beyond anchoring mornings, evenings and administrating, help make simple self-care rituals second nature any time of day. Weave in practices boosting resilience.

Daily Vitamins and Medications – Set a recurring phone alert choosing the time you're most likely home. Keep supplies visible on the counter.

Make Your Bed – This small act creates a sense of order to start the day and represent self-care.

Drink Herbal Tea – Keep a variety of calming teas stocked. Sip mindfully when feeling anxious or needing comfort through the day.

Step Outside – Even 5-10 minutes outdoors in the fresh air and nature resets mood and energy.

Practice Gratitude – Keep a running gratitude list via journal or app of all life's blessings big and small. Add to it often.

Move Body – Take frequent movement breaks when studying or working long hours. Do yoga flows, dance, walk laps or stretch.

Read Uplifting Materials – Fill spare time with inspiring books, podcasts or videos that feed your spirit and refill mental reserves.

Write Down Thoughts – Empty mental clutter onto paper through stream of consciousness journaling or digital voice transcribing apps.

Talk to Friends – Chat about highlights, funny moments and positive news from the day. Social connection boosts oxytocin.

Unplug – Build in device-free blocks focusing on real world engagement. Digital detox time alleviates overwhelm.

Weave self-care into the fabric of everyday life consistently. Even small nurturing actions compound making coping reserves feel fuller.

Infusing Fun and Connection Into Schedules

While structure provides needed scaffolding, an excessively rigid existence breeds burnout. Help your partner balance obligations with fun outlets expressing their spirit. Routines shouldn't feel confining.

Explore building in regular opportunities for:

- Creative pursuits like art, music, DIY projects based on their unique interests. Schedule hobby time.

- Outdoors immersion through gardening, exercising outdoors, hiking, swimming for mood boosts.

- Socializing through standing shared dinners, activity nights, volunteering as a group etc to prevent isolation.

● Adventure infusions via mini weekend road trips, festivals, museums, concerts. Look forward to escapades.

● Game nights, movies and reading times for lighthearted laughter and mental rest. Humor heals.

● Spontaneity reservoirs by allowing **???zero plan zones???** in the calendar open to impromptu fun.

Routines feel most sustainable when they balance obligations with enthusiasm. Protect space for your partner's passions. Delight breeds resilience to endure challenges. With flexibility, consistency comforts rather than confines.

Preparing For High-Risk Times

Staying consistent with healthy routines proves most difficult during high-stress periods like holidays, travel, grief or transitions. Anticipate these demand surges proactively.

Holiday Hustle – During hectic seasons, delegate added tasks to family to reduce stress pileup. Keep up day-to-day routines despite busyness.

Pre-Travel Planning – Before trips account for medication/supplements needing packing, airport accommodations if hyperactivity is an issue, and general sensory-friendly gear to simplify outings.

Grief Support – In times of trauma or loss, connect with grief counseling, support groups, and hotlines as added resources alongside routine self-care.

Major Life Changes – When moving, changing jobs, having kids, etc plan extra special care like mindfulness practices and consistent sleep to stay grounded amidst even positive transitions.

No matter the scenario, identify 1-2 absolutist daily rituals like nourishing breakfasts, brief workouts, meditative tea times to maintain normalcy as an anchor. Keep driving towards baseline health habits between the disruptions.

Thriving Together Through the Chaos

Establishing consistent routines empowers your partner to feel in control when PCOS and ADHD so often make life feel helter-skelter. But know there will be messy beautiful days when schedules go off the rails. Meet each one with compassion.

On mornings when you both sleep through alarms, laugh it off and spontaneously grab breakfast out at a cafe. When plans derail, embrace spontaneity as an adventure. And if Focus just won't come some days despite best efforts, simplify obligations without self-judgment.

Progress happens in a winding path of two steps forward, one step back. As long as you're each moving in a generally positive trajectory, small setbacks just reveal areas for more patience and self-love.

At the end of the day, remind your partner their worth never depends on perfect compliance with routines. They are already enough. Your unwavering support is the safety net to keep trying as life unpredictable life keeps coming. Together, build pockets of peace amidst the chaos.

Daily Routines: Creating Structure for Better Mental Health

When your mind and body feel chaotic and unpredictable from the symptoms of PCOS and ADHD, solid daily routines provide ballast. They act as dependable rituals restoring some sense of control. Amidst the turbulence, routines steady the ship. Even simple consistent habits build mental resilience protecting against crashes. Let's explore practical strategies for deliberately crafting routines that enhance confidence, focus, self-care and connection. Regularity creates space for joy within the daily grind.

Morning Rituals That Jumpstart Intention

Mornings set the stage for each day. A thoughtful, soothing start fuels productivity and eases the transitions ADHD brains struggle with. Make beginning on calm footing priority one.

Hydrate – Drink a full glass of water immediately upon waking to rehydrate and kickstart digestion and focus. Dehydration derails cognition.

Stretch – Take a few minutes for gentle yoga or light calisthenics to get blood moving. This releases muscle tension and boosts energy.

Meditate – Sit quietly observing deep breaths or do a short guided mindfulness exercise before digital stimulation. Grounding clarifies intentions.

Nourish – Eat a balanced breakfast with protein, smart carbs and healthy fat. It prevents later crashes from sugary carbs alone.

Prepare – Lay out clothes, pack bags, and gather belongings by the door the night before avoiding morning scrambling.

Connect – Share an affectionate hug, kiss or check-in with your partner. Start the day immersed in love.

Review Goals – Look over your schedule and make a short list of must-accomplish priorities to set focused intentions.

When mornings feel rushed, everything feels uphill. Commit to routines honoring your holistic needs as worthy of time. The tone you set propels the hours ahead.

Evening Wind-Downs for Restful Sleep

Just as intentional mornings breed balance, purposeful evening routines improve sleep, productivity, and mental reset. Make unplugging a priority, not just collapsing into bed.

Unwind - Spend the last stretch of your commute home listening to music or an audiobook. Separate from work mentally.

Change Clothes - Put on cozy loungewear and set aside electronics and work materials. Signify home as a restful space.

Connect - Chat or cuddle with your partner about your days. Share gratitude. Foster intimacy outside the bedroom.

Unplug - Power down screens at least an hour before bedtime. Blue light delays melatonin release critical for sleep.

Hydrate - Drink water steadily in the evenings to optimize overnight hydration and hormone balance.

Bathe - Take a warm bath or shower to rinse away the day's stress and facilitate relaxation. Add Epsom salts.

Read - Spend quality time with a book, magazine or Kindle. Engaging but easy content calms the mind.

Reflect - Journal about the day's events, lessons and emotions. Empty mental clutter onto paper.

Prepare – Set out tomorrow's outfit, pack bags, and review your schedule and to-do list tonight.

Honoring rest primes your mind, body and spirit for an energized tomorrow. Protect sleep consistency no matter how busy life gets. Even small habitual shifts create big compound benefits.

Weekly Planning for Organization

While consistent daily routines breed stability, you also need bigger picture organization. Take time weekly for proactive planning to reduce mental clutter and anxiety. Get centered.

Coordinate Calendars – Compare work schedules, appointments, kids' activities etc. Record obligations in one master family calendar.

Meal Plan – Draft nutritious dinner ideas and grocery list for the week ahead. Prep components in advance when possible.

Map Goals – Identify 1-3 major priorities to focus on. Schedule blocks on your calendar to designate work time.

Schedule Self-Care – Plug in activities nourishing your mind, body and spirit so they claim time in your week.

Administer Finances – Review budget, pay bills, balance accounts. Automate payments when possible.

Clean and Declutter – Straighten spaces and purge excess possessions creating a resetting sense of calm.

Connect with Support – Note any social outings, therapy appointments, or group activities offering community.

Prepare – Do laundry, tidy rooms, and get supplies/items needed for the upcoming week. Run errands.

When you thoughtfully orchestrate the week ahead, reacting gives way to acting with intention. You frontload focus proactively instead of just responding. Everything flows easier.

Anchoring Your Days In Gratitude

Cultivating daily gratitude practices helps anchor overwhelming days with uplifting perspective and meaning. Make thankfulness part of morning and evening rituals. Studies confirm it boosts mood and resilience.

Keep a Journal – Date each daily entry listing things you feel grateful for – loved ones, comforting items, accomplishments, freedoms, health. Notice the blessings.

Give Thanks Out Loud – Around the dinner table or during morning routines, have family members share aloud one thing that day they feel grateful for. Verbalizing amplifies the power.

Write Thank You Notes – Pen heartfelt cards to people who uplift you expressing what you appreciate about them. The messages brighten their day too.

Savor Your Senses – Pause periodically to mindfully engage your senses fully. Notice details you overlook like birdsongs, fragrances, and breeze on skin. Give thanks for sensory gifts.

Appreciate Challenges – Recognize how adversity and mistakes often guide growth. Be grateful for the grit developed and lessons gained.

Gratitude grants perspective lifting the spirits even during periods of greatest hardship. When incorporated daily, it grounds against spiraling rumination. Count blessings over burdens.

Cultivating Daily Movement and Exercise

Regular exercise provides a critical antidepressant, focus boosting, and stress-relieving outlet benefiting both mental and physical health. Make consistent movement routines non-negotiable.

Start Small – Don't let all or nothing thinking deter starting. Even 10-15 minutes of activity daily like walking, gentle yoga or light weights reaps huge mood benefits. Building up over time feels more sustainable for those managing health conditions.

Pair Activity with Socializing – Plan workouts with friends, family or colleagues. Social motivation helps consistency, and connection protects mental health.

Schedule It – Just like other obligations, reserve time for exercise on your calendar. Treat movement as an essential appointment, not an afterthought.

Make It Fun – Incorporate novelty, games or friendly competition into routine workouts. For example, create treasure hunts on walks, race friends on spin bikes, play "workout bingo" cards mixing exercises.

Multitask – Fold in activity wherever plausible like walking meetings, using stationary bikes or treadmill desks, doing squats during commercial breaks or lunges while brushing your teeth.

Try Different Modalities – Mix up cardio, weights, Pilates, boxing, barre, sports etc. Variety prevents boredom while targeting fitness holistically.

Focus on Feelings – Track not just calories burned but the emotional lift regular movement brings – reduced stress, boosted energy, improved body confidence and self-care pride.

Even modest physical activity every day stimulates feel-good neurotransmitters, circulation, and healthy inflammation balance easing both PCOS and ADHD symptoms. Make it priority self-care.

Relaxation Techniques for Anxiety Relief

While exercise helps physically release tension, purposeful relaxation practices restore mental calm. They curb anxiety and racing thoughts sabotaging focus and sleep. Try different modalities:

Breathwork – Spend 5-10 minutes twice daily consciously deep breathing. Inhale fresh energy, exhale out toxic thoughts. Slow mindful breath regulates the nervous system.

Body Scans – Lie down and gradually turn attention to each area of the body from toes to head noticing sensations. Release tension through each section.

Yoga – Gentle flowing sequences, passive restorative postures, and final savasana meditation elicit relaxation. Match yoga style to your energy level.

Meditation – Sit quietly and focus on the present moment, letting thoughts float by without attachment. Apps provide guided meditations on themes like gratitude or self-love. Start with just 5 minutes.

Visualization – Picture calm imagery like floating on clouds or resting by the ocean. Make visualizations multi-sensory incorporating smells and sounds.

Muscle Relaxation – Alternately tense and relax different muscle groups. Notice the sensations of releasing tightness. Apps provide step-by-step guidance.

Nature Immersion – Spend time outdoors absorbing the soothing negative ions, sunlight, greenery and sounds. Try forest bathing, walking labyrinths, or sitting by water.

Soothing Hobbies – Do calming activities like knitting, coloring, gardening, playing instruments, photography or crafts. Arts and crafts remove mental clutter.

Essential Oils – Place a drop of lavender, bergamot, chamomile or cedarwood oil on your wrists and temples. Inhale the aroma therapeutic properties.

Give yourself permission to prioritize stillness. Protecting your peace empowers productivity, presence, and pleasure long-term. Carve out daily space for quiet mind-body rejuvenation.

Optimizing Time with Loved Ones

Don't let busy schedules or technology creep minimize precious time with your partner, kids or close friends. Prioritize meaningful social connection as a self-care foundation. Loneliness breeds poor mental health.

Schedule It – Block out designated date nights or coffee dates on your calendar to safeguard bonding. Treat quality time as seriously as other obligations.

Take Tech-Free Days – Periodically have 24 hours without technology immersing fully in family activities. Remove distractions.

Share Gratitude – Before bed, have each family member thank another for a kindness, lesson, or happy memory they provided that day. Nurture appreciation.

Ask Meaningful Questions – Rather than default superficial conversations, ask thoughtful questions to more deeply understand each other's needs and goals. Go beyond surface.

Practice Generosity – Do kind acts simply to make your loved ones smile like leaving encouraging notes, cooking their favorite meal or dropping off a favorite treat or gift card at work for them.

VOLUNTEER TOGETHER – Giving back as a family unites everyone in purpose larger than busy lives. Find causes aligned with your passions.

Prioritize One-on-One Time – Ensure you connect individually with each family member's unique needs outside group settings. They'll cherish the undivided attention.

The greatest mental health booster remains consistent intimacy. Set aside distractions to truly see, nourish, protect, and enjoy those who matter most.

Establishing Soothing Bedtime Rituals

Restorative sleep proves foundational for wellbeing. Make evenings purposefully relaxing to set the stage for sound slumber. Little habitual bedtime wind-downs tell the body and brain to rest.

Power Down Screens – Turn off phones, tablets, computers and TVs at least an hour before bed. Blue light hinders melatonin release.

Have a Tea Ritual – Savor a warm cup of chamomile, passionflower or other herbal tea to relax and hydrate.

Write in Gratitude Journal – Jot down 3-5 things that day you feel grateful for. It resets perspective on a high note.

Practice Brief Meditation – Listen to a 10-minute audio body scan or mindfulness meditation to drift off more serenely.

Read Uplifting Books – Curl up with an inspiring memoir, devotional or light fiction. Allow words to wash worries away.

Take a Bath – Soak in warm Epsom salt water scented with lavender essential oil and play soft music. Let stress melt.

Diffuse Sleep Scents – Place a drop of lavender, cedarwood or ylang ylang oil in your diffuser. Breathe in sleep-promoting aromas.

Make Lists – Pour mental clutter onto paper - tomorrow's to dos, weekly goals, grocery needs. Then rest knowing it's captured.

Stretch and Breathe – Flow through gentle yoga poses and pranayama breathing to release physical and mental tension before bed.

When evenings nurture you fully, sleep becomes the sweet ending you wake eager for more of. Protect rejuvenation to handle each day with resilience and joy.

Day by day, simple consistent habits profoundly shape wellbeing, productivity, perspective and relationships. While initially routines feel tedious, their compound benefits over time can't be overstated. What's truly overwhelming is the ceaseless chaos of unstructured days.

Approach organizing routines not as rigid boxes constraining free spirit, but as loving wisdom guardrails protecting your peace. Allow imperfection. Progress flows steadily through commitment to small repeated actions over time, not massive immediate overhaul.

With your partner, design sustainable structures honoring your unique personalities and values. Where attention goes, energy flows. When intention guides your hours, you direct time rather than let it passively direct you.

Reclaim agency amidst the turbulence through purposeful regimens woven into the fabric of each day.

Emotional Support: Being the Pillar Without Being Overwhelmed

Partners of those managing chronic health conditions often naturally fall into the role of steadfast emotional pillar holding the relationship strong when times get tough. However, absorbing the perpetual storms of distress your loved one faces risks depleting your own reserves over time, leading to resentment. How do you balance bearing their burdens with setting boundaries around emotional capacity? Let's explore strategies for providing support, cultivating self-care, and getting help when needed. Your empathy must come from a well of energy that you actively replenish.

Validating Their Emotional Experiences

The first step lies in truly accepting the spectrum of emotions your partner expresses stemming from their dual diagnoses – including the dark, messy ones like anger, hopelessness, or grief. Avoid trying to immediately "fix" painful feelings. Just be present.

Rather than defending or explaining away their symptoms when emotions run high, pause to listen and understand. Ask what thoughts underlie the feelings to deepen insight about their inner world.

Reflect back what you hear without judgment and with empathy:

"I know how upsetting and discouraging managing these symptoms must feel each day."

"This anger is coming from a place of pain about the effects you didn't ask for."

"You have every right to mourn the way this condition has disrupted the joys you imagined for life."

"I can't fully grasp what it's like in your shoes, but I appreciate you helping me understand."

Let them fully express their authentic feelings. Emotional acceptance provides the safety for hope to ultimately emerge amid the darkness. Suppressing their challenges for sake of positivity only breeds distance.

Offer tangible help navigating the emotions. Suggest healthy outlets like journaling, support groups, counseling or complementary therapies to aid processing. Help schedule these self-care respites which replenish their inner well.

When they're caught in storms of lament and self-criticism, gently redirect to recall previous examples of resilience or wins. Help counterbalance discouraging narratives with hope.

Finding Calm in Chaos Together

In the eye of distress and uncertainty their diagnoses trigger, your peaceful presence steadies. Help cultivate daily anchors of calm and meaning amidst the chaos which throws equilibrium off.

Schedule quality time together pursuing activities that build connection and lift spirits - making meals, being in nature, enjoying shared hobbies, volunteering for causes you care about.

Practice stress-relieving rituals as a couple like meditating, massaging one another or soaking in epsom baths. Don't underestimate simple pleasures.

Keep a gratitude list of all blessings big and small. Reciting these gifts and accomplishments when darkness looms restores perspective.

Remind them their value is never defined by productive output. Help release the pressure to handle everything flawlessly. Progress over perfection matters most.

Work together to reduce sources of negative stress and activity overload. Evaluate if obligations deplete more than uplift. What demands can be dropped or delegated?

When they apologize for needing extensive support, reply "I'm always here to help shoulder the rough patches. We support each other no matter what."

Reframe setbacks as opportunities to problem solve together versus reasons to berate themselves. Maintain a spirit of "us versus the issue, not each other."

Your unwavering belief in their abilities to overcome and thrive carries them through stormy seas, back to sanctuary. Hold fast to hope.

Setting Healthy Boundaries Around Your Limits

Being an unconditional emotional pillar for your partner does require boundaries so you don't sacrifice your own needs and wellbeing. Burnout prevents truly being present. Know your capacity and communicate limits sensitively.

If constantly hearing solely negatives starts weighing you down, gently redirect the conversation:

"I want to be your safe space to vent so you don't hold this all in. At the same time, staying stuck in problem focus amplifies despair. Could we balance discussions about some of the hopeful aspects too?"

"My spirit feels drained today. Can we connect by cooking together or watching a comedy instead of processing more worries right now?"

When requests for support become unrealistic, offer compromise:

"I wish I could join every doctor appointment to take notes, but my work schedule makes that really tough. What if we recorded visits on our phones so I can be involved from home?"

"I know how frustrating parenting is some days with the ADHD challenges. I'm happy to take over mornings before work. But let's plan who handles which times to avoid me burning out."

If criticisms about your support approach feel overly harsh, express your feelings while reaffirming commitment:

"I feel hurt when my efforts to help are met with criticism or irritation. But I'm still here. Let's talk through better ways I can show up."

"When every solution I suggest gets rejected, I start taking it really personally. Can you help me understand what doesn't feel supportive so I can modify my approach?"

"I know you lash out at me when you're in pain. But I ask that you find ways to vent anger that don't attack my character."

You can lovingly safeguard your emotional needs while remaining engaged. Measure out compassion in sustainable chunks. Your partner will benefit most from a present peaceful you, not a depleted shell.

Helping vs Enabling

It's natural to want to intervene solving every struggle your partner faces. But in your eagerness to assuage their troubles, take care not to inadvertently enable unhelpful behaviors or thinking patterns. The healthiest support empowers their autonomy.

For example, completing tasks on their behalf when frustration mounts often provides short-term relief but deprives them of opportunities to build skills managing ADHD symptoms independently. It's a slippery slope between helping and enabling dependency.

Similarly, rushing to soothe every worry and self-criticism stops them from learning tools to self-regulate emotions and inner negative chatter. Don't immediately solve problems they're fully capable of handling themselves.

You walk the line between being loving assistant and possessive enabler. Have patience letting your partner struggle productively through challenges building their own coping muscles and earned confidence.

The most empowering support scaffolds just enough – helping them devise systems for self-organization, gently nudging them to start difficult conversations themselves, role modeling healthy thinking patterns through your lived example.

Master the art of holding back unsolicited advice while still providing safety nets. Offer support that props them up rather than holds them back. Help your partner learn to fly solo even if the process feels bumpy. The falls make the flying sweeter.

Relinquishing Control Over Their Treatment Journey

One of the greatest acts of love is letting your partner steer their own health journey. Avoid playing authoritarian doctor. While your input adds helpful perspective, their diagnoses ultimately impact their lived experience most. Allow autonomy over managing care.

Respect their right to start and discontinue medications or specific diets on their own terms even if you fervently disagree. Different treatments affect you as the partner far less directly. Make suggestions not demands.

If new approaches seem to deteriorate their condition, kindly share your observations then let them come to their own conclusions when ready. People more fully embrace change when self-directed.

Support their treatment choices even if very different from what you would select. Their path to thriving may veer away from the conventional at times. Keep an open mind.

Let your role be an unconditional listening ear they can fully be themselves around, not a parental enforcer. They show up best for healing when self-motivated versus pressured to please you.

The most empowering partners adopt a "You lead, I support" mentality regarding this journey that isn't yours to control. Your unwavering faith in their inner wisdom provides the safety net to keep trying new roads until answers unfold.

Managing Stress Around the Unknowns

The uncertainty chronic health conditions breed often overwhelms loved ones. Fears arise not knowing if or when new symptoms may flare or progress.

Tolerating ambiguity feels excruciating. However, anticipating hypothetical worst cases wastes present moments. Manage worries through:

Mindfulness - Get out of future spiral thoughts by paying attention to right now - sights, sounds, sensations. Breathe slowly. Take in the stillness and stability surrounding temporary health storms.

Perspective - When your mind leaps to catastrophic "what ifs" about decline or debility, balance those with factual realities about the patient, stable condition your partner currently enjoys. Counter-balance anxiety with logic.

Presence - Rather than endlessly researching obscure risks online, redirect attention to tangible actions of loving service you can focus on day-to-day like preparing nourishing meals or organizing medication refills. Active care alleviates worry.

Release - Journal stream of consciousness style allowing yourself to vent every pinned up fear and frustration to release their grip. Then burn or shred the pages. Let imagined outcomes go.

Meaning - Get involved with communities supporting your partner's condition to see the incredible hope, resilience and purpose that arises even facing challenges. Surround despair with meaning.

Your calmness anchors your partner's worries. Manage your own stressors consciously so they don't compound an already full emotional load. Breathe through fears of the unknown, so now feels peaceful.

Supporting Other Relationships Impacted

Finally, recognize your partner's diagnoses may strain broader family dynamics and friendships when misunderstandings arise or limitations feel unclear. Play a mediating role educating loved ones.

If parents, siblings or friends make thoughtless comments clearly hurtful to your partner, pull them aside privately later to provide perspective:

"Kelly doesn't resist family events to be anti-social. Crowds and noise just get really overwhelming with her sensory issues. Can we help adjust group gatherings to be more ADHD friendly for her?"

"Rob isn't shirking work responsibilities. You have to understand ADHD executive functioning and focus challenges make his job much harder. Let's have some compassion about the disability he wrestles with."

"Her mood swings don't mean she doesn't love you. PCOS hormones and pain wear on anyone. She needs support, not judgment."

Offer to share educational resources to promote empathy and bridge rifts.

Remind loved ones progress is often incremental. Make space for their learning curve aligning with your partner's health journey. With gentle guidance, transform relationships into healing sources instead of added burdens.

Protecting Your Own Wellbeing Needs

You cannot indefinitely pour from an empty pitcher. Ensure caring for your partner doesn't consume your whole identity and reserves. Honor your own stress limits and self-care needs too.

Take Time Off - Regularly schedule mini-breaks like weekends away or evenings out to emotionally recharge. You return better equipped to support.

Set Communication Boundaries - If constant venting becomes draining, gently redirect to solution focus. Also limit electronic intrusions after work hours.

Ask For Help - Call on family, friends or hire help with household obligations when your load feels unmanageable. Delegate tasks.

Therapy Helps - Seek counseling to process your own stress, sadness or relationship struggles. You cannot guide someone else through depths you haven't navigated.

Join Support Groups - Connect with others caring for partners with your loved one's diagnoses. Shared experiences provide comfort.

Pursue Passions - Stay engaged in hobbies, sports, faith community and other outlets feeding your spirit outside the relationship.

Practice Mindfulness - Spend time tuning into your emotions and needs through meditation, journaling, nature sitting or chanting. Don't just power through.

You remain the most vital caregiver when you first care for yourself. Protect your light by setting healthy impermeable emotional and practical boundaries. Your partner wishes you well-rested and at peace.

Seeking Solutions Together

Managing the unpredictable ups and downs of chronic health conditions tests even the strongest relationships. But with team spirit, creativity and forgiveness, every chaos spell also represents an opportunity to deepen care and commitment. You are on the same side combating external forces, not each other.

Rather than resenting your partner's limitations, ask "How can we adapt and improvise so these diagnoses impact our daily life less?" Maybe that means family helps out with household duties or you delegate junior work roles. If intimacy gets sidelined by fatigue, get creative exploring new ways to connect and pleasure each other. When social events become overwhelming, turn date nights into quiet game nights in.

Of course acknowledge grief, frustration and mourning over lost dreams or Independence. But don't settle there. Keep mining your partnership for solutions viewing circumstances through a lens of possibility, not defeat. If one path closes, you widen another. As long as you cling to hope together, you will weather the storms in time.

Finally, appreciate that as many valleys as this journey brings, the peaks of profound purpose, character, closeness, and celebration it breeds soar higher. Your compassion muscle develops strength. Hardships reveal sources of unexpected grace. Dark clouds prepare you to relish the light. Cherish your partner for the resiliency and grit these roads have revealed. You signed up for all of life's complexity and beauty when you committed your hearts as one. This experience deepens gratitude for every breath shared. Keep seeking hope.

Daily Routines: Creating Structure for Better Mental Health

When your mind and body feel erratic and unpredictable from the symptoms of PCOS and ADHD, establishing solid daily routines provides ballast. They act as dependable rituals restoring some sense of control. Amidst the turbulence, routines steady the ship. Even simple consistent habits build mental resilience protecting against crashes. Let's explore practical strategies for deliberately crafting routines that enhance confidence, focus, self-care and connection. Regularity creates space for joy within the daily grind.

Morning Rituals That Jumpstart Intention

Mornings set the stage for each day. A thoughtful, soothing start fuels productivity and eases the transitions ADHD brains struggle with. Make beginning on calm footing priority one. I've mentioned a lot of these before, but it just stands repeating. Repetition builds remembering.

Hydrate – Drink a full glass of water immediately upon waking to rehydrate and kickstart digestion and focus. Dehydration derails cognition.

Stretch – Take a few minutes for gentle yoga or light calisthenics to get blood moving. This releases muscle tension and boosts energy.

Meditate – Sit quietly observing deep breaths or do a short guided mindfulness exercise before digital stimulation. Grounding clarifies intentions.

Nourish – Eat a balanced breakfast with protein, smart carbs and healthy fat. It prevents later crashes from sugary carbs alone.

Prepare – Lay out clothes, pack bags, and gather belongings by the door the night before avoiding morning scrambling.

Connect – Share an affectionate hug, kiss or check-in with your partner. Start the day immersed in love.

Review Goals – Look over your schedule and make a short list of must-accomplish priorities to set focused intentions.

When mornings feel rushed, everything feels uphill. Commit to routines honoring your holistic needs as worthy of time. The tone you set propels the hours ahead.

Evening Wind-Downs for Restful Sleep

Just as intentional mornings breed balance, purposeful evening routines improve sleep, productivity, and mental reset. Make unplugging a priority, not just collapsing into bed.

Unwind - Spend the last stretch of your commute home listening to music or an audiobook. Separate from work mentally.

Change Clothes - Put on cozy loungewear and set aside electronics and work materials. Signify home as a restful space. I would also recommend this after arriving home from work, it is amazing how just changing clothes can make you feel about what you are doing, or going to do.

Connect - Chat or cuddle with your partner about your days. Share gratitude. Foster intimacy outside the bedroom.

Unplug - Power down screens at least an hour before bedtime. Blue light delays melatonin release critical for sleep.

Hydrate - Drink water steadily in the evenings to optimize overnight hydration and hormone balance.

Bathe - Take a warm bath or shower to rinse away the day's stress and facilitate relaxation. Add Epsom salts. I would also recommend a warm/hot shower, followed by a few minutes under cooler (if not cold) water.

Read - Spend quality time with a book, magazine or Kindle. Engaging but easy content calms the mind.

Reflect - Journal about the day's events, lessons and emotions. Empty mental clutter onto paper.

Prepare – Set out tomorrow's outfit, pack bags, and review your schedule and to-do list tonight.

Honoring rest primes your mind, body and spirit for an energized tomorrow. Protect sleep consistency no matter how busy life gets. Even small habitual shifts create big compound benefits.

Weekly Planning for Organization

While consistent daily routines breed stability, you also need bigger picture organization. Take time weekly for proactive planning to reduce mental clutter and anxiety. Get centered.

Coordinate Calendars – Compare work schedules, appointments, kids' activities etc. Record obligations in one master family calendar. My wife and I have our Google Calendars synced with each other. Though sometimes she'll look at her calendar and see some Continuing Education I have going on and ask who the task belongs to.

Meal Plan – Draft nutritious dinner ideas and grocery list for the week ahead. Prep components in advance when possible.

Map Goals – Identify 1-3 major priorities to focus on. Schedule blocks on your calendar to designate work time.

Schedule Self-Care – Plug in activities nourishing your mind, body and spirit so they claim time in your week.

Administer Finances – Review budget, pay bills, balance accounts. Automate payments when possible. My wife and I have started a monthly event we call a Budget Party to do this. We hate doing it, but by calling it a party, it makes it seem more fun than it is.

CLEAN AND DECLUTTER – Straighten spaces and purge excess possessions creating a resetting sense of calm.

Connect with Support – Note any social outings, therapy appointments, or group activities offering community.

Prepare – Do laundry, tidy rooms, and get supplies/items needed for the upcoming week. Run errands.

When you thoughtfully orchestrate the week ahead, reacting gives way to acting with intention. You frontload focus proactively instead of just responding. Everything flows easier.

Anchoring Your Days In Gratitude

Cultivating daily gratitude practices helps anchor overwhelming days with uplifting perspective and meaning. Make thankfulness part of morning and evening rituals. Studies confirm it boosts mood and resilience.

Keep a Journal – Date each daily entry listing things you feel grateful for – loved ones, comforting items, accomplishments, freedoms, health. Notice the blessings.

Give Thanks Out Loud – Around the dinner table or during morning routines, have family members share aloud one thing that day they feel grateful for. Verbalizing amplifies the power.

Write Thank You Notes – Pen heartfelt cards to people who uplift you expressing what you appreciate about them. The messages brighten their day too.

Savor Your Senses – Pause periodically to mindfully engage your senses fully. Notice details you overlook like birdsongs, fragrances, and breeze on skin. Give thanks for sensory gifts.

Appreciate Challenges – Recognize how adversity and mistakes often guide growth. Be grateful for the grit developed and lessons gained.

Gratitude grants perspective lifting the spirits even during periods of greatest hardship. When incorporated daily, it grounds against spiraling rumination. Count blessings over burdens.

Cultivating Daily Movement and Exercise

Regular exercise provides a critical antidepressant, focus boosting, and stress-relieving outlet benefiting both mental and physical health. Make consistent movement routines non-negotiable.

Start Small – Don't let all or nothing thinking deter starting. Even 10-15 minutes of activity daily like walking, gentle yoga or light weights reaps huge mood benefits. Building up over time feels more sustainable for those managing health conditions. Use timers! Our house has four Alexa devices and the odds are high that one of them has a timer or alarm going on at any given time. As I'm writing this, there's an alarm going off, so that I, the "neuro-typical one" can make the most of my lunch break. After a session of writing, I will take the dog out, and then grab a quick bite to eat, and go back to work. If you are the neuro-typical one, these things can help you as well.

Pair Activity with Socializing – Plan workouts with friends, family or colleagues. Social motivation helps consistency, and connection protects mental health. Even something as simple as a dog walking group can create paths for socializing, both for you, your partner, and your dog!

Schedule It – Just like other obligations, reserve time for exercise on your calendar. Treat movement as an essential appointment, not an afterthought. If it isn't on the schedule, it may not happen.

Make It Fun – Incorporate novelty, games or friendly competition into routine workouts. For example, create treasure hunts on walks, race friends on spin bikes, play "workout bingo" cards mixing exercises. If you're driving, make a game out of seeing how many of a specific type of car you can find. My wife and I recently had a five hour drive in which we counted how many different types of Toyota Rav4s we could see. It was around 500, split between at least two body styles. No, Toyota did not pay me to mention that.

Multitask – Fold in activity wherever plausible like walking meetings, using stationary bikes or treadmill desks, doing squats during commercial breaks or lunges while brushing your teeth. Or, you know, fold laundry during commercial breaks or during meetings, especially if you don't need your camera on.

Try Different Modalities – Mix up cardio, weights, Pilates, boxing, barre, sports etc. Variety prevents boredom while targeting fitness holistically.

Focus on Feelings – Track not just calories burned but the emotional lift regular movement brings – reduced stress, boosted energy, improved body confidence and self-care pride.

Even modest physical activity every day stimulates feel-good neurotransmitters, circulation, and healthy inflammation balance easing both PCOS and ADHD symptoms. Make it priority self-care.

Relaxation Techniques for Anxiety Relief

While exercise helps physically release tension, purposeful relaxation practices restore mental calm. They curb anxiety and racing thoughts sabotaging focus and sleep. Try different modalities:

Breathwork – Spend 5-10 minutes twice daily consciously deep breathing. Inhale fresh energy, exhale out toxic thoughts. Slow mindful breath regulates the nervous system.

Body Scans – Lie down and gradually turn attention to each area of the body from toes to head noticing sensations. Release tension through each section.

Yoga – Gentle flowing sequences, passive restorative postures, and final savasana meditation elicit relaxation. Match yoga style to your energy level.

Meditation – Sit quietly and focus on the present moment, letting thoughts float by without attachment. Apps provide guided meditations on themes like gratitude or self-love. Start with just 5 minutes.

Visualization – Picture calm imagery like floating on clouds or resting by the ocean. Make visualizations multi-sensory incorporating smells and sounds.

Muscle Relaxation – Alternately tense and relax different muscle groups. Notice the sensations of releasing tightness. Apps provide step-by-step guidance.

Nature Immersion – Spend time outdoors absorbing the soothing negative ions, sunlight, greenery and sounds. Try forest bathing, walking labyrinths, or sitting by water.

Soothing Hobbies – Do calming activities like knitting, coloring, gardening, playing instruments, photography or crafts. Arts and crafts remove mental clutter.

Essential Oils – Place a drop of lavender, bergamot, chamomile or cedarwood oil on your wrists and temples. Inhale the aroma therapeutic properties. To me, the best is to have the lavender in the diffuser while sipping lavender chamomile tea.

Give yourself permission to prioritize stillness. Protecting your peace empowers productivity, presence, and pleasure long-term. Carve out daily space for quiet mind-body rejuvenation.

Optimizing Time with Loved Ones

Don't let busy schedules or technology creep minimize precious time with your partner, kids or close friends. Prioritize meaningful social connection as a self-care foundation. Loneliness breeds poor mental health.

Schedule It – Block out designated date nights or coffee dates on your calendar to safeguard bonding. Treat quality time as seriously as other obligations. If you do not think to schedule time with friends and loved ones, they may not happen.

Take Tech-Free Days – Periodically have 24 hours without technology immersing fully in family activities. Remove distractions. Talk.

Share Gratitude – Before bed, have each family member thank another for a kindness, lesson, or happy memory they provided that day. Nurture appreciation.

Ask Meaningful Questions – Rather than default superficial conversations, ask thoughtful questions to more deeply understand each other's needs and goals. Go beyond surface.

Practice Generosity – Do kind acts simply to make your loved ones smile like leaving encouraging notes, cooking their favorite meal or dropping off a favorite treat or gift card at work for them.

Volunteer Together – Giving back as a family unites everyone in purpose larger than busy lives. Find causes aligned with your passions.

Prioritize One-on-One Time – Ensure you connect individually with each family member's unique needs outside group settings. They'll cherish the undivided attention.

The greatest mental health booster remains consistent intimacy. Set aside distractions to truly see, nourish, protect, and enjoy those who matter most.

Establishing Soothing Bedtime Rituals

Restorative sleep proves foundational for wellbeing. Make evenings purposefully relaxing to set the stage for sound slumber. Little habitual bedtime wind-downs tell the body and brain to rest.

Power Down Screens – Turn off phones, tablets, computers and TVs at least an hour before bed. Blue light hinders melatonin release.

Have a Tea Ritual – Savor a warm cup of chamomile, passionflower or other herbal tea to relax and hydrate.

Write in Gratitude Journal – Jot down 3-5 things that day you feel grateful for. It resets perspective on a high note.

Practice Brief Meditation – Listen to a 10-minute audio body scan or mindfulness meditation to drift off more serenely.

Read Uplifting Books – Curl up with an inspiring memoir, devotional or light fiction. Allow words to wash worries away.

Take a Bath – Soak in warm Epsom salt water scented with lavender essential oil and play soft music. Let stress melt.

Diffuse Sleep Scents – Place a drop of lavender, cedarwood or ylang ylang oil in your diffuser. Breathe in sleep-promoting aromas.

Make Lists – Pour mental clutter onto paper - tomorrow's to dos, weekly goals, grocery needs. Then rest knowing it's captured.

Stretch and Breathe – Flow through gentle yoga poses and pranayama breathing to release physical and mental tension before bed.

When evenings nurture you fully, sleep becomes the sweet ending you wake eager for more of. Protect rejuvenation to handle each day with resilience and joy.

Day by day, simple consistent habits profoundly shape wellbeing, productivity, perspective and relationships. While initially routines feel tedious, their compound benefits over time can't be overstated. What's truly overwhelming is the ceaseless chaos of unstructured days.

Approach organizing routines not as rigid boxes constraining free spirit, but as loving wisdom guardrails protecting your peace. Allow imperfection. Progress flows steadily through commitment to small repeated actions over time, not massive immediate overhaul.

With your partner, design sustainable structures honoring your unique personalities and values. Where attention goes, energy flows. When intention guides your hours, you direct time rather than let it passively direct you. Reclaim agency amidst the turbulence through purposeful regimens woven into the fabric of each day.

Beyond Medications: Lifestyle Changes for Dual Diagnosis Harmony

While prescription treatments provide vital relief helping manage chronic health conditions, truly optimizing wellness requires an integrative approach. Certain supportive lifestyle measures can profoundly improve PCOS and ADHD symptoms when used consistently.

However, radical overnight transformations often backfire. Gentle incremental steps feel more sustainable. Have patience fine-tuning a lifestyle rhythm that nurtures body, mind and spirit holistically. Let's explore evidence-based changes together you can make around nutrition, movement, sleep, stress relief, and organization. What you do day-to-day is just as powerfully medicinal as any pill when practiced with care over time.

Harnessing the Power of Nutrition

Diet proves foundational because food provides the basic biochemical building blocks shaping hormones, neurotransmitters, and every bodily process. Optimizing nutrition assists nearly all aspects of PCOS and ADHD management. However, there's no universally ideal "PCOS and ADHD diet." Find gentle aligned nourishment that works best for you.

Avoid Extremes – Any plan too restrictive or complicated inevitably fails long-term. Don't attempt dramatic exclusions without medical guidance. Progress flows from adding in more wholesome foods, not just eliminating "bad" ones.

Lower Glycemic Load – Focus on foods that release sugar into the bloodstream slowly through high fiber, protein and fat. This helps stabilize blood sugar and insulin. Enjoy quality carbs from whole grains, starchy vegetables, legumes, and some fruits.

Increase Produce – Eat a rainbow of vegetables and moderate fruits each day. Produce provides antioxidants, prebiotics, fiber, and anti-inflammatory benefits. Herbs and spices add flavor and nutrients.

Pick Lean Proteins – Protein foods aid concentration, satiety, and muscle tissue repair. Include plant proteins like nuts, seeds, beans, lentils alongside organic poultry, eggs, fatty fish, and yogurt. Avoid processed deli meats. Salmon is great in this regard.

Choose Healthy Fats – Incorporate fatty acids like olive oil, avocado, nuts, seeds, and salmon to control inflammation and balance hormones. Avoid trans fats and limit saturated animal fats.

Stay Hydrated – Drink enough water between meals to stay hydrated. Signs like fatigue, sugar cravings, and mental fog signal underhydration exacerbating symptoms. Herbal tea and sparkling water offer variety.

Manage Portions – Overeating strains hormones, metabolism, and cognition. Using smaller plates and mindful eating help maintain portions without deprivation mentality.

Keep Snacks Handy – Pack grab and go snacks like nuts, veggies, hard boiled eggs, fresh fruit, and yogurt to prevent energy crashes or impulsive unhealthy purchases.

Minimize Alcohol – Alcohol dysregulates neurotransmitters and hormones. Heavy drinking worsens aspects of both conditions. Have occasional moderate portions focusing on red wine, clear liquors, and low sugar mixers.

Caffeinate Wisely – While shown to boost focus and alertness in ADHD, excess caffeine stresses the adrenals worsening anxiety. Keep intake moderate and avoid past noon.

Supplement Selectively – Discuss specific supplements that support hormonal balance, cognition, and metabolism with your healthcare team based on labs and symptoms. Quality matters. Start low doses and monitor effects.

Patience, flexibility, and teamwork help discover nourishing staples benefitting your bodies long-term. Support each other's intentions with compassion. What you do consistently matters more than perfection.

The Benefits of Regular Movement and Exercise

Alongside nourishment, regular physical movement provides a powerful medicine for bodies and minds managing PCOS and ADHD. The benefits are bountiful from better weight management to improved sleep, focus, stress resilience, confidence and energy. Make activity a non-negotiable daily priority.

Start Small and Make It Fun – Even short 10-15 minute workouts 4-5 times weekly reap huge gains. Choose activities you genuinely enjoy from dancing to kayaking so it feels like play, not punishment. Bringing fun fuels consistency.

Incorporate Strength Training – In addition to cardio, include light weights, resistance bands, or bodyweight exercises. Building muscle boosts metabolism, hormones, and intrinsic motivation from seeing progress.

Try High Intensity Interval Training (HIIT) – Alternating intense bursts with recovery periods trains the body efficiently with less time commitment. Apps offer guided HIIT options requiring minimal equipment.

Multitask Movement – Take frequent physical activity breaks when studying or working. Do chair yoga, stretch, walk outside or climb stairs. Build rewards like episodes of a favorite show contingent on completing exercise.

Spark Your Cardio – Activities like jogging, swimming, jumping rope, and spin classes strengthen your heart and lungs while flooding the body and brain with feel-good endorphins that boost mood and energy. Find what you most enjoy.

Optimize Your Time – Identify pockets of time allowing consistent movement like morning energizers, lunch break walks or before-dinner workouts. Integrate exercise into your schedule rather than leaving it as an afterthought.

Make It Social – Plan workouts with friends, partners, small groups or fitness meetups. Social motivation improves consistency, and human connection nurtures mental health.

Track Non-Scale Victories – Beyond pounds, note benefits like better sleep, balanced energy, less pain, positive outlook, and self-confidence growing through movement. Celebrate fitness as self-care.

With compassionate consistency, exercise becomes therapeutic, not punishing - a celebration of what your body can achieve. Prioritize daily movement meditatively. You would be surprised by how much simply owning a dog helps with so much of those items I just mentioned.

Optimizing Sleep Quality and Habits

With the fatigue and insomnia accompanying PCOS and ADHD, quality sleep rarely comes effortlessly. However, restorative rest proves foundational for physical and mental health. Test different strategies to improve your sleep efficiency. Protect prioritizing slumber.

Set a Sleep Schedule – Keep bed and wake times consistent including weekends. Routines trigger the brain's sleep-wake homeostasis regulating hormones and circadian rhythms.

Optimize Sleep Hygiene – Keep the bedroom cooler, dark, and quiet. Finish eating 2-3 hours before bed. Limit alcohol and caffeine after 2pm. Remove screens and stressful clutter from the space.

Wind Down Before Bed – Spend the 90 minutes before bed reading, stretching, meditating or listening to calm music to transition into drowsiness. Unplug from electronic stimulation.

Try Restorative Yoga and Breathwork – Gentle centering yoga poses and breathing exercises reduce racing thoughts making space for relaxation. If restless, try alternate nostril breathing or exhale lengthening.

Take Warm Baths – Warm water cues body temperature changes initiating sleep hormones while easing muscle tension. Add Epsom salts and calming essential oils like lavender.

Use Sleep Supplements Judiciously – Ask your doctor about short-term melatonin, magnesium glycinate, or theanine if insomnia persists. They help recalibrate natural sleep-wake cycles. Avoid long-term dependency.

Nap Strategically – Limit napping to 20-30 minutes to avoid disrupting nighttime sleep. However, brief power naps improve focus, mood, and alertness.

Keep a Sleep Diary – Note daily bedtime, wake time, sleep quality, lifestyle factors impacting rest, and sense of daytime alertness. Patterns inform solutions. Share with your doctor.

Prioritize troubleshooting sleep consistently. Without solid rest, managing complex health challenges feels infinitely harder. Protect rejuvenation for the long haul.

Mastering Stress Resilience Techniques

Since chronic stress significantly exacerbates both PCOS and ADHD, calming skills provide essential tools in your toolkit. Restoring nervous system equilibrium through mindfulness, breathwork, andifestyle choices alleviates anxiety and promotes level-headedness.

Establish a Practice – Try short 5-10 minute daily sitting meditation focusing on the breath and present moment mindfulness. Silencing mental chatter builds focus muscles overtime. Apps provide guided sessions.

Walk in Nature – Spend time outdoors consciously absorbing the sights, smells and sensations. Nature is healing. Even urban green spaces reduce anxiety. Try forest bathing, hiking, or sitting by water.

Breathe Deeply – Consciously take longer fuller inhales and extended complete exhales. Deep diaphragmatic breathing switches the body into rest-digest mode.

Try Grounding – Cue your senses into the present when stress spirals through visualization, holding a comforting tactile object, or noticing your feet's physical connection to the floor.

Do Tai Chi and Yoga – Their flowing movements synchronize breath, body and focus in the present moment. Follow along with online videos.

Diffuse Calming Scents – Scents like lavender, chamomile, cedarwood and bergamot reduce anxiety and improve sleep when used in aromatherapy.

Listen to Body Rhythms – Slow down and tune into your natural cycles of sleepiness, hunger, and energy to maximize cognitive functioning aligned with biological needs.

Identify Stress Triggers – Track situations, thoughts or interactions that typically trigger worry and agitation. Then consciously work to modify or limit those stressors.

Counseling Helps – Therapists teach invaluable skills for resilience when managing perceived threats and uncertainties. Make stress management a regular session focus.

Don't underestimate small centering practices weaving calm throughout days. Reduce unnecessary frenzy in schedules where possible. Your inner stability ripples out.

Building Executive Functioning Skills

Since ADHD involves deficits with executive functioning, you can help strengthen mental focus, organization, time management, and impulse control by regularly practicing key skills. fortify these cognitive muscle groups.

Establish Routines – Anchoring each day with consistent morning, evening, and self-care rituals provides structure lacking internally. Routines build habits gradually.

Timebox Focus – Set a timer for 25-30 minute blocks of distraction-free work time with 5 minute breaks between them. Gradually extend focus stamina avoiding burnout.

List Priorities – Each morning, define a short manageable list of must-accomplish items to prioritize the most important one or two tasks. Don't get derailed veering off-list.

Single Task – Choose just one priority task to devote your full attention to until reaching a logical stopping point. Bouncing between many half-completed projects breeds mental clutter.

Remove Distractions – Turn off phones, email, and closing office doors to minimize interrupting high-priority cognitive work. Noise cancelling headphones also help.

Use Tools – Timers, alarms, whiteboards, paper planners, electronic calendars and to do apps provide needed scaffolding. Identify systems you'll actually use consistently.

Start Small – Don't get discouraged when focus wavers or organizing systems get derailed. Expect setbacks and imperfections when building new skills. Just resume patiently.

Reward Progress – Praise yourself for focus stamina achieved, clutter conquered, or tasks completed. Small gains build intrinsic motivation. Celebrate neuroplastic change.

With compassionate consistency, you can rewire thought patterns and habits promoting executive function gains. Be your own loving coach through progress and pitfalls.

Harnessing the Power of Counseling and Community

Finally, don't underestimate the psychological support routinely connecting with therapists and community provides. While lifestyle and medical management help day-to-day, counseling and peers fill emotional needs.

Counseling teaches vital coping skills – Work with a counselor versed in positive psychology, CBT techniques, mindfulness, and social/emotional needs associated with your dual diagnoses. Even during stable times, therapy nurtures growth and resilience. Schedule regular appointments.

Group support alleviates isolation – Join in-person or online groups to share experiences and resources for ADHD, PCOS, chronic conditions, LGBTQIA+ support, etc. You are not alone on this journey. Connect with those who most intimately understand your experience.

Spiritual engagement breeds meaning – If faith community and practices anchor you, stay involved to nourish spiritual wellbeing. If not, seek uplifting secular communities focused on service, charity or social change that give your days purpose.

Therapy aids communication skills – Couples counseling helps you and your partner healthily communicate needs, collaborate on lifestyle changes, and navigate tensions constructively. Don't wait until serious issues arise to get support.

Coaching builds habits – Work with an ADHD coach on motivation, time management, maintaining routines, and combining lifestyle changes. Their structured assistance keeps you progressing.

Practice self-compassion – Be your own best cheerleader. Recognize that setbacks and struggles relate to symptoms, not inadequacy. You have all you need inside to keep growing.

With compassion, accountability, and wisdom from supporters who deeply understand your experience, you feel empowered consistently moving forward with hope.

Sustaining Progress Through Ups and Downs

Implementing major lifestyle changes presents inevitable ups and downs. Some days new regimes feel invigorating, other days completely unmanageable. Expect flows and ebbs along this winding path of insight.

Stay patient with yourself and your partner through occasional backsliding. Hold lapses compassionately without judgment. One comfort binge or week of forgotten supplements means nothing in the big picture.

Celebrate small daily actions demonstrating commitment to wellbeing - a short walk, drinking more water, taking a rest day from work. Build self-trust through showing up for your needs consistently, even imperfectly.

When progress lags, avoid punitive reactions. Ask what barriers feel most challenging right now and restrategize your approach. There are always periods of stagnation, confusion and regrouping when growing.

Share the journey with peers facing similar ups and downs. Their camaraderie and wisdom helps you gain perspective during pitfalls and valleys. With support, inspiration returns.

Most importantly, frame lifestyle changes as manifestations of self-love, not punishment. Choose adaptations allowing sustainable nourishment of body, mind and spirit. What gently helps you thrive? This is a process of nurturing your whole being.

While the road holds twists, turns and detours, you hold the power to steer your days with care. Even small steps forward gain momentum when consistently nurtured. Trust the process.

Planning for the Future: Fertility, Pregnancy, and Parenting Challenges

For couples navigating life with PCOS and ADHD, contemplating future parenthood often stirs up many questions and concerns. From fertility obstacles to pregnancy health risks to worries about coping with an ADHD child, proactively educating and planning reduces fears of the unknown.

While everyone's journey proves unique, insight from experts and others' experiences equips you to tackle hurdles along the way. With teamwork, creativity and support, you can thoughtfully grow your family in alignment with your dreams. Let's explore proven strategies for maximizing fertility prospects, ensuring a healthy pregnancy, and parenting effectively with ADHD.

Overcoming PCOS Fertility Challenges

Due to chronic ovulation problems, PCOS often interferes with easy conception. However, many fertility treatments prove effective helping couples conceive. Patience and medical guidance are key. Don't lose hope.

Track ovulation – Kits detecting luteinizing hormone surges in urine combined with basal body temperature tracking maximize chances by timing intercourse precisely. Apps synthesize data.

Improve egg quality – Supplements like myo-inositol, coenzyme Q10, and melatonin support quality egg maturation. But check with a reproductive endocrinologist before taking new supplements.

Try ovulation induction medication – Drugs like clomiphene stimulate regular ovulation in most women. If ineffective after 3-4 cycles, explore injectables like FSH inducing multiple eggs per cycle. Risks like multiples exist.

Know when to seek help - Consult a reproductive endocrinologist if under 35 and unable to conceive after 6 months of well-timed intercourse or over 35 after 6 months of unsuccessfully trying. Time matters.

Get screened – Ask your ob-gyn for thorough testing needed – bloodwork, HSG dye test, and semen analysis. Identify any obstacles aside from simply anovulation like blocked tubes or low sperm count requiring alternate treatments.

Consider insemination – Intrauterine insemination (IUI) inserts concentrated sperm directly into the uterus, bypassing cervical mucus challenges some PCOS women have. When paired with ovulation drugs, success rates are good.

Weigh IVF pros and cons – In vitro fertilization combining egg retrieval and sperm in a lab dish to create embryos for implanting in the uterus proves successful for many. But it also involves costs, medication demands, and risks requiring discussion.

Evaluate surgery options – Laparoscopic ovarian drilling is sometimes used short-term to stimulate ovulation when other options fail. Discuss thoroughly given lower success rates long-term.

Lean on community – Connect with in-person and online groups for support during the emotional fertility treatment process. You don't journey alone.

Patience, hope, and seeking multiple professional opinions provides key reassurance throughout your fertility journey. Stay anchored in self-care and partnership.

Maximizing Odds of a Healthy Pregnancy

Once pregnant, maintaining healthy habits protects mom's wellbeing and baby's development. Planning ahead aids in navigating inevitable PCOS pregnancy challenges.

Monitor glucose – Insulin resistance raises gestational diabetes risk requiring glucose checks and possibly medication. Follow provider guidelines for ideal control.

Supplement Folate - Start prenatal vitamins with methylfolate form before conception because PCOS elevates neural tube defect risks. Use throughout pregnancy.

Manage weight – Discuss optimal pregnancy weight gain and diet with your OBGYN. Steady increases prevent large spikes in blood sugar. Spread intake evenly.

Reduce inflammation – An anti-inflammatory diet emphasizing produce, lean proteins, fiber and healthy fats prevents flares worsening PCOS. Stay active to lower oxidative stress.

Treat anxiety and depression – Seek counseling to process pregnancy emotions. Discuss any preexisting mental health medication needs with your psychiatrist. Many options are low risk.

Watch for preeclampsia –Elevated blood pressure and protein in urine indicating preeclampsia is more common with PCOS. Report concerning symptoms like swelling immediately.

Prepare for early delivery – Due to heightened risks like preeclampsia and diabetes, many providers induce labor or schedule C-sections for PCOS pregnancies around week 37-38. Plan accordingly.

Get progesterone support – Since PCOS causes sluggish progesterone rise, doctors often prescribe suppositories preventing miscarriage. Use as directed.

Connect with community – Join online groups discussing PCOS pregnancy for advice and comfort from others overcoming similar hurdles. You are not alone.

While greater attentiveness proves important, thousands of women with PCOS successfully deliver healthy babies every day. Stay hopeful reading their encouraging stories. Monitor changes closely and lean on your care team.

Cultivating Coping Skills for ADHD Parenting

ADHD parenting presents unique rewards and challenges. Certain strategies help nurture your child's strengths while minimizing behavioral struggles:

Educate yourself – Read parenting books, take courses, and absorb podcasts or YouTube channels on ADHD parenting specifically. Insights prevent self-blame.

Foster strengths – Nurture their creativity, empathy, humor, spirit of adventure, media talents like making videos, and any passionate interests through activities, mentorships and unstructured play time.

Establish structure – Balancing flexibility with routines provides needed security. Have consistent waking, meals, homework, family time, and bedtimes without rigidity.

Simplify directions – Break requests into clear step-by-step instructions. Have child repeat each part back. Checklists and timers help them work independently.

Manage stimulation – Notice situations triggering restlessness like noisy crowds, interrupting siblings, or too many play options. Adjust environments proactively preventing overwhelm.

Teach coping skills – Role model and guide breathing exercises, quiet time alone, talking through frustrations, and healthy outlets like exercise releasing impulsive energy.

Avoid shaming – Don't label their differences as naughty or defiant behavior worthy of punishment. Empathize with ADHD struggles requiring unique parenting adaptations.

Find support – Connect with counselors, parenting coaches, support groups and respite care assisting ADHD families. You don't need to figure everything out alone.

Practice self-care – Make time for your own stress relief outlets like friendships, hobbies, and counseling. Monitor feelings of isolation, burnout or depression.

While uniquely challenging at times, embracing your child's neurodiversity gifts breeds connection. With mindfulness and self-care, both you and your child thrive.

Making School Accommodations for ADHD Kids

Important conversations and plans ensure your ADHD child gets the classroom support they require. Don't assume the school naturally provides appropriate assistance.

Get evaluated – Ask your child's pediatrician for a cognitive assessment determining any learning disabilities or ADHD requiring an IEP or 504 plan detailing legally mandated accommodations.

Share the report – Provide the full evaluation detailing their unique needs to the principal, teachers and special education coordinator. Highlight key recommended accommodations.

Request periodic meetings – Set up IEP review sessions every 6 months where your child's providers can attend and explain needs to all staff involved in their education and progress monitoring.

Involve administrators – Alert principals directly anytime significant bullying, stigma or teacher friction occurs so leadership can help resolve conflicts quickly.

Learn your rights – Understand disability protections in your state so you can cite violations requiring correction. Familiarize yourself with special education laws.

Communicate needs – Inform teachers ahead of field trips or stimuli-heavy days that adjustements preventing sensory overload help your child learn. Suggest fidget toys, noise cancelling headphones, preferential seating etc.

Track progress – Keep all report cards, progress reports, evaluation results, disciplinary records etc. to discern needed academic support adjustments each year.

Shift support – If certain accommodations prove ineffective, request modifications or assistance like small group instruction or counseling. Meet your child's changing needs.

With proactive partnering and compassionate resolve, school can provide a safe, supportive haven for your child to gain independence and self-esteem.

Medicating Children with ADHD

If optimal school and home modifications don't sufficiently help your child's focus and self-regulation challenges, ADHD medications present another option in close provider guidance.

Whenever I think about ADHD and children, I always think about my father, who was never anything near being a doctor, but his medical diagnosis for ADHD was, "It's not real, it's just kids being kids. Attention deficit and hyperactivity? That's the definition of a child." Fortunately, I did not have ADHD and live with a science denier, like I'm sure many people did (and possibly still do, unfortunately). Fortunately, science has progressed far enough that we can now regulate the symptoms in children, but even then, be careful not to overdo things.

Go slowly – Medications help many kids transform their abilities, but they're not the first or only recourse. Try environmental changes, therapy skills and parenting strategies first.

Get evaluated – Seek testing by a pediatric psychiatrist experienced in childhood ADHD to formally confirm diagnosis since some symptoms overlap with other conditions like autism.

Learn formulations – Research stimulant and non-stimulant options to make informed choices about potential effectiveness and side effect risks requiring monitoring.

Start low – Once prescribed, begin with the lowest dose spanning at least a month to observe changes and tolerance before considering increases. Document symptoms.

Time strategically – Many parents administer meds on school days and skip weekends and breaks to allow "drug holidays" preventing dependence. Discuss benefits/drawbacks of this approach with your psychiatrist.

Watch reactions – Note any appetite, sleep, mood or behavioral changes and communicate closely with your child and doctor about optimizing meds based on reactions. Expect gradual fine tuning.

Re-evaluate annually – Have your child's providers assess prescribing indications, proper dosing and still-needed accommodations every school year as needs evolve developmentally.

Don't over rely – Medication assists functioning but doesn't substitute for parenting, lifestyle choices, or skill building needed long-term. Use it as one component, not the sole intervention.

While uniquely challenging at times, embracing your child's neurodiversity gifts breeds connection. With mindfulness and self-care, both you and your child thrive.

Making School Accommodations for ADHD Kids

Important conversations and plans ensure your ADHD child gets the classroom support they require. Don't assume the school naturally provides appropriate assistance.

Get evaluated – Ask your child's pediatrician for a cognitive assessment determining any learning disabilities or ADHD requiring an IEP or 504 plan detailing legally mandated accommodations.

Share the report – Provide the full evaluation detailing their unique needs to the principal, teachers and special education coordinator. Highlight key recommended accommodations.

Request periodic meetings – Set up IEP review sessions every 6 months where your child's providers can attend and explain needs to all staff involved in their education and progress monitoring.

Involve administrators – Alert principals directly anytime significant bullying, stigma or teacher friction occurs so leadership can help resolve conflicts quickly.

Learn your rights – Understand disability protections in your state so you can cite violations requiring correction. Familiarize yourself with special education laws.

Communicate needs – Inform teachers ahead of field trips or stimuli-heavy days that adjustments preventing sensory overload help your child learn. Suggest fidget toys, noise cancelling headphones, preferential seating etc.

Track progress – Keep all report cards, progress reports, evaluation results, disciplinary records etc. to discern needed academic support adjustments each year.

Shift support – If certain accommodations prove ineffective, request modifications or assistance like small group instruction or counseling. Meet your child's changing needs.

With proactive partnering and compassionate resolve, school can provide a safe, supportive haven for your child to gain independence and self-esteem.

Maintaining Your Relationship and Wellbeing

Amidst the demands of parenting, prioritizing self-care and couples' time protects family health. You must nourish your foundation first.

Connect daily – Schedule quality time together ritualistically, even if brief. Chat over coffee, take walks, play board games as a family. Don't let parenting always center kids.

Trade off self-care – Alternate "me time" where one parent gets a morning off or weekend day to rejuvenate while the other handles the kids. You both deserve outlets.

Utilize family help – Accept offers from grandparents to babysit allowing date nights and short couple getaways. Community parenting prevents isolation.

See a counselor – Seek therapy addressing parenting struggles proactively before chronic issues develop. Learn skills to avoid burnout and talk through tensions.

Tackle stress – Make relaxation practices like exercise, meditation, massage and supportive friendships pillars in your routine. Lower daily pressure when possible.

Get creative – Improvise bonding rituals that nourish intimacy like showering together, exchanging handwritten love notes, enjoying weekly at-home date nights when childcare proves difficult.

Forge patience – When parenting woes test your bond, recall shared values and grit to overcome any hurdle side-by-side with good faith. This too shall pass.

Protecting your foundation equips you to weather parenting storms through creativity, flexibility and forgiveness. Your children's sense of security stems from your modeled relationship. Prioritize caring for the caregivers.

Embracing the Unexpected Blessings

However you envision your pregnancy unfolding or family expanding, life often brings surprises forcing us to let go and trust unfolding mysteries. Parenting becomes a journey without scripts or assurances. But staying open allows profound meaning to enter when plans rearrange.

Throughout each twist and turn - from adapting fertility tactics when challenged to embracing an exceptional ADHD child's gifts – maintain belief in possibilities beyond what you can see.

Your child arrives exactly as meant to, in the right timing, even when health hurdles or detours delay the expected path. With support and self-compassion, you ably handle all that this profound privilege of nurturing young lives entails.

Building a Supportive Network: Surrounding Yourselves with Positivity

Living with chronic health conditions like PCOS and ADHD poses unique challenges mentally, emotionally, and practically. While your partnership provides the primary pillar of strength, cultivating a diverse support network proves invaluable long-term. Community breeds resilience on difficult days. Let's explore strategies for surrounding yourselves with uplifting people and finding your tribes. With wisdom, care and camaraderie binding you, the path looks brighter.

Leaning on Family and Friends

Begin building community among those already dear to your lives but who require education regarding your health journeys. Offer to share helpful articles and books that provide perspective. Convey specific ways loved ones can uplift and assist at pivotal times.

Share Supportive Content – Send family and friends informative yet positive articles and social media accounts illuminating life with your diagnoses. Increased insight breeds empathy.

Be Open About Your Experience – Give candid glimpses into your reality via social media vulnerably showing tough days along with triumphs. Let loved ones into your world.

Explain Your Needs – Tell trusted confidants how they can practically assist on especially demanding days – childcare, meals, cleaning help, transportation etc. People want guidance for helping.

Ask About Their Lives – While needing support yourself, also reciprocate interest in your loved ones' lives. Mutual care bonds relationships. Listen attentively.

Allow Imperfection – Remember friends and family cannot always relate or respond perfectly. Focus on intentions over delivery. Tolerating missteps cultivates grace.

Cultivate Quality Over Quantity – Invest in family and friends bringing most nourishment, even if that means pruning draining relationships. Protect your emotional space.

Coordinate Practical Help – Use online tools like meal trains or care calendars so friends can sign up assisting with tasks like providing dinner or rides when health flares.

With openness, generosity and compassion on all sides, cherished people provide nurturing community. While they can't fully grasp your challenges, their loyal love still carries you through.

Finding Your People Through Support Groups

One of the greatest gifts you can discover is sharing your journey with others living with the same diagnoses. Mutual understanding breeds instant connection. There are many groups to explore:

ADHD Support Groups – Locate in-person and online groups specifically for adults managing ADHD. Both general coed and women's groups exist locally and virtually. The deep sense of togetherness provides comfort.

PCOS Support Groups – Connect with women-centered groups and online communities focused on all aspects of navigating PCOS – medical, emotional, reproductive etc. Shared stories prove healing.

Dual Diagnosis Groups – Search for support communities uniquely devoted to the intersection of ADHD and female hormonal disorders. Individual stories speak your language.

Chronic Illness Groups – Wider chronic condition communities for issues like depression, anxiety, autoimmunity and more offer solidarity if you don't locate ADHD/PCOS specific groups locally. We all need empathy.

Special Interest Groups – Join groups bonding over meaningful causes and activities – religious study, charities, fitness meetups, book clubs, hobby message boards. Build meaningful relationships beyond just diagnoses.

While family loves you unconditionally, nothing replaces finally feeling "normal" and instantly understood among those walking similar paths. Find your people and your place to fully be yourselves.

Connecting with PCOS and ADHD Bloggers/Influencers

Along with in-person community, virtual voices on social media deliver inspiration you can tap into anytime needing motivation or hope on lonely days. Follow influencers who uplift and educate.

Seek Role Models – Follow people thriving with your conditions who offer positivity and practical tips across platforms like Instagram, TikTok, YouTube, and their own blogs. Let their stories propel you.

Learn the Science – Follow doctors, nurses, therapists and researchers sharing the latest medical developments and healthy living strategies for PCOS, ADHD and dual diagnoses. Stay updated.

Broaden Perspective – Diversify the viewpoints you take in across ages, backgrounds and stages. Single moms, couples starting careers, LGBTQ+ community, women navigating menopause - everyone offers wisdom.

Note Red Flags – Be aware of accounts breeding fear, exaggerating struggles without solutions, making sweeping claims about miracle cures or dismissing medicine. Take advice with a grain of salt.

Find Your Joy-Spreaders – Favor positive voices celebrating self-care wins, body acceptance, neurodiversity gifts and releasing comparisons. Consume media uplifting your spirit.

Participate In Discussions – Engage actively in account posts and Lives. Comment with your own experiences, questions and inspiration to cultivate community.

Digital voices become cherished companions reminding you of shared humanity when your path feels lonely. Let their triumphs and truths walk beside you.

Bonding with Partners On The Journey

One of the most comforting resources you can lean on is other couples navigating these diagnoses too. Their lived partnership insights and empathy often outdo professional guidance alone. Try:

Pairing with a Mentor Couple – Ask a provider or support group facilitator if an experienced couple might mentor you. Having their seasoned perspective offers reassurance.

Joining Partner Support Groups – Search for couples support groups focused on thriving with dual diagnoses. Shared laughs and wisdom get you through the uphill climbs.

Participating in Retreats – Attend small group retreats for couples managing ADHD and other conditions. Often held in nature, they combine nurturing workshops with bonding.

Meeting Other Power Couples – When you encounter inspiring partners giving talks or on panels, make a point to approach them afterward. Ask to stay in touch.

Coaching Each Other – If both you and another couple seek coaching, offer to be each other's accountability partners between sessions. Check in regularly.

Following Other Couples Online – Find blogs, videos and accounts where partners share their lessons learned navigating the tumultuous and beautiful. Take comfort in the glimpses of teamwork.

Chatting Candidly with Friends – Bond with couple friends you trust over shared relationship challenges, milestones, and victories across life stages. Leaning on community never stops.

While every couple's path proves unique, encouragement from those who intimately understand your dynamics delivers hope on days you feel alone. Shared humanity heals.

Seeking Out Wellness Practitioners

Alongside emotional support, expand your network of wellness professionals able to address the layered physical and mental health components of dual diagnoses. They offer expertise bridging the gap between standard and alternative care.

- Naturopathic Doctors (NDs) – These holistically-minded physicians combine medical training with nutrition, herbs, supplements and lifestyle counseling attuned to root causes and prevention. Their integrative lens assesses care options through a cooperative team approach.

- Integrative Nurse Practitioners – These advanced practice nurses take a whole person approach to care weaving together standard treatments, alternative modalities like essential oils and mindfulness, health coaching support and naturopathic protocols based on your values and needs.

- Functional Medicine Providers – This new generation of practitioners focuses on addressing core imbalances and optimizing wellbeing through nutrition, minimally invasive testing, genomic analysis, detoxification, stress management, and targeted supplementation. Their emphasis lies in collaboratively treating root causes and the whole system.

- Health and Wellness Coaches – These professionals guide clients in reaching health goals through motivation, accountability, meal planning assistance, lifestyle design mentorship, and making purposeful sustainable behavior changes. They empower you as drivers of your own care.

Seek out practitioners receptive to complementary approaches and honoring your innate wisdom about your bodies. Assemble your own personalized team catering to all dimensions of health.

Exploring Faith Communities

If spirituality plays a strong role grounding you, don't underestimate the gift faith communities can provide, both in tangible help and emotional healing. However, finding the right fit may take some searching.

Consider Your Needs – Reflect on what you hope to gain – acceptance, counseling services, rituals/practices, volunteer opportunities, children's programming, diversity, etc. Then look for groups aligned with your priorities.

Give it Time – Don't expect instant comfort. It takes patience finding where you belong. Try various congregations or groups within the same religion before judging fit. Stay open.

Have a Consultation – Schedule an intro call with a prospective clergy member to discuss your spiritual journey and health challenges. Ensure integration and support feel feasible.

Connect Directly – Introduce yourselves to welcoming members after services. Explicitly share your conditions and any accommodations that would aid participation.

Reach Out Privately – If a faith leader ever makes stigmatizing statements about disabilities or non-nuclear family structures, discretely but directly address the impact such messaging bears. Education breeds change.

Consider Your Dealbreakers – If certain faith communities philosophically misalign with your values or worldview, seek those embracing diversity, neurodiversity, mental health, and modern families. Find your people.

While not right for everyone, for those so inclined, spiritual community can profoundly help make sense of challenges through sacred connection. Where you feel seen and secure, wisdom flows.

Cultivating Your Chosen Family

Beyond biological family, intentionally nurture a "chosen family" of kindred spirits who become like siblings. They don't replace relatives, yet provide bonds uniquely resonating.

Look for friends who:

- Uplift and inspire you to grow in positive ways

- Show up for you during life's ups and downs

- Accept and appreciate the real, messy you - differences and all

- Share your values, passions and quirks

- Make you laugh until it hurts

- Offer the gift of mutual vulnerability and support

- Remain loyal through time, distance and circumstances

This handpicked community becomes your refuge and rock reminding you that you don't walk alone. Their unconditional understanding fills places where bio family may fall short. Surround yourself with those who feel like home.

Safeguarding Your Inner Sanctuary

While community nurtures mental health, also know your limits and keep inner circles reasonably sized. Too many demands on time and empathy drain reserves. Check in on whether relationships energize or tax you. Reduce points of stress protecting inner calm.

Gently say no to taking on support roles beyond your emotional capacity - volunteering, extensive childcare, sitting on boards etc. You must care for yourself first before filling other cups.

Limit time with consistently negative contacts breeding drama, judgment, or excessive venting. Politely decline if certain social events feel depleting versus replenishing. You teach people how to treat you by what you permit.

Let go of toxic bonds out of obligation. Relationships should uplift both parties the majority of the time. If consistently one-sided or strained, wishing someone well from a distance may better honor your peace.

Fill life instead with positive influences across modalities - therapists, authors, spiritual leaders, friends, community programs – whatever breeds motivation, balance and progress. Then radiate that light.

By proactively surrounding yourselves with empathy, care, inspiration and expertise, you weave a web of support mitigating challenges. While pacing proves important, recognize too that giving and receiving community often fills your cup exponentially more than it drains. Let the right people love you through the journey.

On days you feel overwhelmed or hopeless, recall you walk in the company of many who have ventured these roads before. Their camaraderie carries you until answers unfold. With compassion within and without, continue moving toward wholeness. The light awaits.

Rediscovering Romance: Keeping the Spark Alive Amidst Challenges

Romantic relationships inevitably evolve through chapters, sometimes drifting into stagnancy or discord along life's unpredictable path. But when dual diagnoses like PCOS and ADHD enter the picture, nurturing an intimate bond often requires even more concerted effort and creativity.

As passions wane and tensions arise, it's common to simply accept this as the new normal. However, by intentionally fostering playfulness, appreciation and persistence, you can rediscover the magic allowing your story to feel exciting at every turn, not just the beginning.

Let's explore ways to rekindle emotional and physical intimacy through hope, understanding and reveling in everyday adventures.

Releasing Expectations and Assumptions

Before reigniting dimmed sparks of romance, first reflect on any rigid assumptions needing release. You hold more power to brighten your bond when you let go preconceived notions of how chemistry and intimacy "should" unfold.

For example, are you judging the quality of your connection by standards like:

- Peak early passion and excitement lasting perpetually

- Consistent sexual desire and functioning

- Emotional stability without rollercoasters

- Agreement on big life decisions

- Interests and social needs staying the same

- Equality in initiation and reciprocation

The reality is that in any relationship, passions ebb and flow, people grow and evolve, and health impacts change dynamics. By embracing this impermanence, you free yourself to reconnect in new ways right where you're at now versus chasing unrecoverable past ideals.

When you release rigid expectations, hope emerges to write a fresh storyline. What matters isn't checking boxes of how relationships "should be" but rather honoring your continually unfolding story. Recommit to each next chapter.

Reawakening Playfulness and Adventure

As domesticity sets in, many couples fall into comfortable routines losing touch with their youthful sense of play, risk-taking, novelty and fun early on. However, you can rekindle lightheartedness again.

Leave notes in surprising places to make your partner smile and feel that giddy excitement of infatuation. Send inside joke texts during the workday. Exchange spontaneous massages or dance breaks. Try new creative date ideas monthly pushing beyond habits.

Fantasize together about dream vacations, homes, or side businesses. Let imagination wander. Doodle or make vision boards capturing future goals that reignite passion. Adult responsibilities needn't extinguish childlike curiosity forever.

When you encounter novel experiences as a couple, it bonds you in exhilaration and laughter deepening history. Uncover hidden parts of your city together. Attempt new restaurants, dancing styles, concerts, classes or sports neither tried before. Allow spontaneity to scatter routine once more.

Your carefree early days don't have to represent the pinnacle of partnership. Write fresh memories daily delighting in each other and the gifts of now. Joy always remains available at any stage when you begin a new chapter.

Releasing The Fairytale Narrative

Many implicitly buy into unrealistic relationship fairytales fueled by media, causing distress when reality proves different. However, embracing imperfections fosters intimacy and grace to weather all seasons.

Rather than seeking a perfect untroubled union, acknowledge challenges as opportunities to practice vulnerability, conflict resolution, creative problem-solving and unconditional commitment.

When friction arises, avoid jumping to conclusions about incompatibility. Friction simply indicates areas needing deeper understanding. Explore what vulnerable conversations and compromises might bridge gaps.

Perfection cannot be sustained long-term. Forgo fantasies about effortless relationships. Instead aim for authenticity - loving in spite of and even because of each other's flaws and differences. Here you find the beauty.

Redefining sensuality beyond physical acts also opens new avenues for closeness. Share self-acceptance, intellectual exchange, laughter, whispered hopes and quiet companionship. This sensuality of soul runs far deeper than any fantasy.

By embracing imperfections, you craft an extraordinary relationship no fairytale glimpsed - a story with richness, wisdom, character and hard-won joy through togetherness.

Maintaining Intimacy Amidst Health Struggles

PCOS and ADHD symptoms inevitably impact couples' intimacy. Fatigue, pain, distraction, differing desires and medication side effects interfere. However, prioritizing ongoing emotional and physical connection breeds resilience through challenges.

Start by communicating openly about your changing needs and limitations to avoid taking fluctuations personally. "I want to be close, but tonight I just can't summon the energy for sex itself. Can we cuddle and talk instead?" When you understand effects aren't rejections, tensions release.

Get creative expanding sensuality definitions beyond traditional sex scripts. Exchange massages, take baths together, read erotic works, try new fantasies, schedule morning intimacy avoiding fatigue. Meet shifting capacities with flexibility, not frustration.

Protect playfulness. Laugh together frequently about the awkwardness of positions gone awry, toppled lubricant bottles killing the moment's sexiness, and comical bodily sounds. Humor lightens sensitivities straining chemistry.

Focus on emotional intimacy - the caring, support, trust and tenderness that builds confidence in the foundation. Verbalize appreciation for each other. Then physical connections flow more smoothly.

When health struggles increasingly isolate partners in solo coping, make concerted efforts bonding through it all - cards, hugs, quick texts conveying you're in their corner. Little gestures build relationship resilience.

Stay patient through phases requiring compromise. The only constant is change. Ups and downs invite you to reinvent intimacy uniquely together, not mechanically mirroring others' relationships. Write your own sensual love story.

Reawakening Admiration and Attraction

Over time, familiarity risks breeding a lack of awe or novelty in relationships. Reigniting admiration involves paying attention to each other's essence versus taking traits for granted:

Look for unnoticed daily actions expressing your partner's deeply caring nature - fixing your favorite snack when you're sad, tidying clutter unprompted when you're overwhelmed, remembering little personal preferences that make you feel special. Notice the little graces.

When you eavesdrop on their conversations or interactions outside your relationship, tune into their shining wit, compassion, wisdom, or playfulness. Hear them as if for the first time.

Take moments to literally gaze at your partner - their lovely eyes, infectious grin, endearing expressions, attractive build - as if seeing them anew. Let the love seep in.

Appreciate out loud overlooked or undervalued attributes you adore like their resilience, creativity, quirky jokes, or how much laughter they bring into your home. Praise strengths beyond surface qualities.

Thank them for stabilizing gifts easily taken for granted - their loyalty through life's unpredictable ups and downs, daily acts of service or comforting routines only they provide.

There is no better aphrodisiac than heartfelt praise. When you focus on your unique reasons for cherishing your partner, old embers reignite. Reveal the extraordinary in their ordinary. This is the alchemy of admiration.

Cultivating Therapeutic Communication

Tensions inevitably arise in relationships, but poor communication patterns turn issues toxic. Promoting openness, understanding and problem resolution keeps conflicts from calcifying into lasting coldness.

Set weekly or biweekly "State of Our Union" check-ins sharing feelings about the relationship proactively before resentments build. Prevent small hurts from quietly amplifying over time.

Learn each other's intended methods of showing love - physical touch, gift giving, quality time, verbal affirmation. Neither style is superior, but mismatch causes disconnect.

When communicating grievances, use gentle "I statements" to claim ownership of feelings versus accusatory "you statements" putting partners on defensive.

Always allow each person uninterrupted time to share their perspective one at a time without impatience. Feeling totally heard defuses reactivity.

Watch that criticisms don't veer into hurtful insults, exaggerations, or contempt. Healthy feedback discusses specific changeable actions, not fixed character attacks.

If tensions escalate unproductively, call a time out to cool down and self-soothe before resuming with clearer heads. Silence or space can heal better than harmful words.

When all seems resolved, seal conversations with hope. Verbalize confidence in your shared abilities to implement compromises, forgiveness and new beginnings.

Communicating with compassion, honesty and openness to understand breed intimacy. Mastering healthy conflict resolution forms the bedrock supporting growth through all seasons of partnership.

Seeking Outside Support

If communication stagnates despite best efforts or chronic frustrations plague your bond, recognize reaching out for professional guidance is wisdom, not weakness. An outside perspective helps recalibrate stuck patterns.

Consider meeting with a therapist who can teach communication tools, provide perspective when you feel stuck in your own narratives, give homework prompting vulnerability, and facilitate navigating difficult topics constructively. Work together identifying areas for growth instead of assigning blame.

For more serious relationship issues, seek counseling specifically focused on reconciliation, trauma healing and emotional needs surrounding chronic illness. Specialists in these areas deliver valuable guidance.

If health struggles increasingly prevent regular quality time together, look into respite care through local programs or in-home health aides to help manage daily responsibilities so you can reconnect. Don't go it all alone.

Lean on community from support groups, other couples navigating similar diagnoses, and close friends exemplifying partnerships you admire. Their wisdom lights the way when your own dims.

You don't have to figure everything out solo. Support makes space for the clarity, tools and hope required to rediscover intimacy. Together you rise stronger.

Nurturing Your Partnership Holistically

Don't let the busyness of life and stress of health conditions crowd out consistently nurturing foundational pillars of your relationship beyond quick fixes. Rejuvenate your shared roots with:

Quality Time – Establish weekly or biweekly dedicated dates, even if just watching movies at home, to intentionally reconnect without distractions.

Physical Touch – Exchange daily non-sexual affection like hugs, hand-holding, foot rubs, and cuddling to stay bonded. Touch conveys care.

Shared Experiences – Make time for adventures and holidays expanding your life stories and inside jokes. New chapters fortify history.

Intellectual Connection – Discuss meaningful ideas from podcasts, books, documentaries and classes. Share shifting perspectives, goals and curiosities keeping your mental intimacy alive.

Sexual Exploration – When able, brainstorm creative ways to enjoy sensual connection like romantic getaways, couples intimacy workshops, boudoir photography, or sex toys to prevent sexual ruts.

Spiritual Grounding – If faith resonates, enjoy spiritual practices together like prayer, worship, yoga, or volunteering through your community. Shared values anchor relationships.

Optimism and Gratitude – Regularly express genuine appreciation for each other's kindnesses, progress and support. Positivity outshines negativity.

Mutual Respect – Always speak to each other with esteem, even during disagreements. Demeaning words bruise bonds. Keep perspective when hurt.

Accountability – Lovingly help each other grow by encouraging healthiest choices while allowing imperfection. Supporting dreams bonds you.

Small consistent investments protecting your foundational wellbeing accumulate exponentially over decades. Nurture that sacred space where your love thrives through all seasons.

Embracing Each Phase with Flexibility

Rather than regretting periods when health or stress strains your romantic life, embrace these phases with compassion. They inevitably come and go. Your control lies in maintaining perspective.

When sexual challenges arise, avoid despairing this as forever your new normal. Explore creative solutions, but let go rigid ideas of how intimacy "should" unfold.

If sparks naturally wane in periods focused on child-rearing, career demands or crisis coping, trust flickers rekindle once daily pressures release. Your history allows faith.

Understand romance often alternates being a priority. When inflows of energy recede for a time, pour attention into nourishing other areas like parenting, friendship, and self-care. Nothing is fixed permanently.

Look at transitions as opportunities to reinvent connection in new ways right where you're at now versus trying to reclaim the past. Meet each other's needs today.

Focus on consistent acts of service, kindness and commitment when former modes of intimacy feel elusive. Your foundation still stands firm.

Through ups and downs, follow love's lead with resilience. Flow with the natural ebb and flow of relationships' tides across the long arc of commitment. What matters most remains.

May you look back on valleys traversed as what ultimately deepened bonds, character and wisdom to see beauty in every phase's purpose. Even fallow periods plant seeds for later abundance.

When past notions of partnership dissolve, bravely face the blank page together now writing a new narrative. Let creativity, not resignation, author each chapter.

Your story exceeds limitations or endings society's scripts dictate. You generate glittering stardust romance with every inside joke, movie night, slow dance in the kitchen and 3am conversation sealed with laughter.

This alchemy emerges whenever you choose to see, touch, share in your partner's essence. Even the longest histories feel exciting when made new by presence.

May you always begin again in each moment, falling into one another with fresh awe. The greatest romances perennially reinvent adventures, passion and treasure buried right underfoot the whole while.

Navigating Perimenopause and Menopause with PCOS and ADHD

⸺

I had not thought about including a chapter on this life stage until my wife mentioned that being perimenopause herself, PCOS would cause strange things to happen outside of what normally happens during menopause. Relax, she isn't going to grow feathers or anything. PCOS really is a thing that affects people their entire lives, even when you would think these kind of things would stop.

As women with PCOS and ADHD transition into their 40s and 50s, the onset of perimenopause and eventual menopause brings new considerations. The hormonal fluctuations and changes during this midlife stage interact uniquely with preexisting endocrine conditions, potentially exacerbating symptoms.

As partners, you play an important supportive role through this transition. Understanding common challenges and creative solutions will help you empathetically embrace this turning point together. With knowledge, lifestyle shifts, compassion and perseverance, you can weather "the change" and uncover liberating possibilities on the other side.

Demystifying Perimenopause

Let's start by clearly defining this extended transition period preceding menopause, which often begins in the late 30s and 40s but lasts several years. Many women mistake perimenopause symptoms as emergence of new health issues rather than natural aging effects.

During perimenopause, the ovaries slowly decrease production of estrogen and progesterone while fertility declines. However, ovulation doesn't fully cease and periods continue during this stretch - although they may be irregular, heavy/prolonged, or missed altogether some months.

The fluctuating and overall dropping hormone levels destabilize menstrual cycles as the body transitions into menopause. Lower estrogen also triggers common effects like hot flashes, sleep disruption, mood swings, vaginal atrophy, and slowed metabolism.

PCOS offers a unique complication. Many women don't realize the periods they had were not true menstruation resulting from ovulation, but rather breakthrough bleeding from hormone withdrawal when progesterone pills or birth control are stopped. So early perimenopause signals can be missed.

Irregular cycles, pelvic pain, and heavy flow due to lack of ovulation are often considered "normal PCOS periods." Watch also for emerging hot flashes, sleep disruption, palpitations, and thinning hair. These distinguish perimenopause.

While the average duration lasts 4-5 years, perimenopause persists anywhere from 2 to 8 years before the onset of menopause. Patience and tracking help discern what changes reflect aging versus preexisting PCOS.

Coping with Compounded Hormone Fluctuations

For women simultaneously navigating PCOS and perimenopause, the double hormone rollercoaster intensifies symptoms like mood, energy, and metabolic issues. Estrogen drops while testosterone persists, setting up a collision.

You may notice your partner's ADHD-related emotional sensitivity and reactivity spike during this time as estrogen plummets. The combined impact of declining estrogen, continuing androgens, erratic ovulation, and life stage pressures prove challenging.

PCOS symptoms like unwanted hair growth, pelvic pain, and cystic acne also frequently worsen entering the 40s before later resolving post-menopause when ovarian function halts. Feelings of grief and resentment often accompany this resurgence.

Cultivating extraordinary self-care prevents double hormone chaos from hijacking mental health. Gentle nutrition, stress relief practices, therapeutic outlets like art and music, and social support provide balance through the volatility when possible.

Lifestyle measures easing other menopause symptoms help perimenopausal PCOS as well:

- Regular exercise for mood/sleep/health

- Yoga and meditation for equanimity

- Supplements like omega-3s and vitamin D

- Minimizing caffeine, alcohol and sugar

- Vaginal moisturizers and lubricants for comfort

- Acupuncture for hormonal regulation

- Positive self-talk and gratitude practices

You play an important role encouraging rest, releasing judgement about limitations, and urging compassionate inner dialogue when your partner's self-critic arises. Your stability braces her during the storm.

Evaluating Supplements and Prescriptions

Certain supplements and medications sometimes help mitigate perimenopausal ups and downs without fully replacing missing hormones the way HT does. Under provider guidance, options to consider include:

Black Cohosh – This herb appears effective reducing hot flashes and night sweats in some women, likely by influencing estrogen receptors. It may also improve mood, sleep, and heart palpitations. However, stay under 6 months to avoid risks.

Antidepressants – SSRIs like citalopram, sertraline and fluoxetine boost serotonin providing non-hormonal relief for depression, insomnia and hot flashes. Discuss risks like low libido with your prescriber.

Gabapentin – This nerve pain medication may also help reduce hot flash intensity and night sweats when used short-term. However, it can cause side effects like drowsiness, dizziness and swelling.

Clonidine – This blood pressure medicine might decrease frequency of moderate to severe hot flashes. However, potential side effects include dry mouth, drowsiness, dizziness and constipation.

Progesterone Cream – Some providers suggest over-the-counter bioidentical creams to provide the progesterone that drops during perimenopause. However, efficacy and safety remain unclear. Use the minimum effective dose if pursuing.

Vitamin E – This antioxidant might offer mild relief from hot flashes, night sweats and disrupted sleep when taken in doses around 800 IU daily. However, check with your doctor about potential interactions.

These interventions may temper effects, but close oversight by all providers ensures safety and modified dosing with your PCOS status. Tracking symptom changes prevents staying on ineffective or harmful supplements long term.

Hormone Therapy Considerations

The most effective medical treatment for relieving troublesome perimenopausal or menopausal symptoms remains hormone therapy (HT). However, with a history of PCOS, additional considerations exist.

The main HT formulations are:

- Estrogen only: Recommended for women without a uterus to avoid endometrial cancer risks

- Progestin plus estrogen: The most common to protect the uterine lining in women still possessing a uterus

- Ovarian hormone therapy: Utilizing DHEA, testosterone and progesterone

While HT nearly eliminates hot flashes, night sweats, and vaginal dryness, it may cause additional unwanted hair growth or acne flares in some PCOS patients due to androgen activity. However, this varies. Monitor changes.

Discuss your partner's unique symptom priorities with their provider. Lower dose estrogen creams or rings may temper side effects. Progestin-only regimens are an option as well.

Many women do well on combination HT managing bothersome menopause effects without PCOS symptom exacerbation. Have open conversations weighing pros and cons of trying hormone therapy or natural supplements.

Keep close tabs on changes if opting to start HT. Follow up regularly with all prescribing practitioners to ensure her full health picture stays in balance. Be alert to any mood shifts suggesting estrogen levels need adjusting.

Emphasize that finding the optimal solution requires patience, diligent tracking of progress and side effects, and continual reassessment as needs evolve. You're on this journey together!

Lifestyle Strategies for Managing Menopausal Changes

While hormone levels largely drive perimenopause and menopause impacts, certain lifestyle measures substantially ease this major life transition:

Focus on Rest – Prioritize adequate nightly sleep, brief daytime naps if needed, and quiet solo time recharging Given the high physical and mental demands of this phase. Don't burn the candle at both ends.

Adapt Fitness Routines – Stay active for emotional and physical wellbeing, but reduce intensity if managing new fatigue Levels. Try yoga, walking, swimming, and light weights. Even short activity spurts help.

Eat Nutritiously – Focus diet on antioxidant-rich colorful produce, plant proteins, fiber and healthy fats that balance blood sugar and hormones. Some find symptom relief reducing gluten, dairy and sugar.

Stay Hydrated – Drink ample water and herbal tea to prevent dehydration contributing to many common symptoms. Carry water reminding yourself to sip regularly.

Dress In Layers – Keep hot flash remedies like portable fans, cold packs, cooling bandanas and extra layers or cover ups handy to swiftly adjust temperature swings.

Tweak Your Space – Maintain bedrooms around 65 degrees with layered bedding you can adjust. Throw off blankets during night sweats. Use moisture wicking sheets and sleep in breathable pajamas.

Carve Out Me-Time – Surround yourself with nurturers like counselors, massage therapists, and friends who lend ears. Prioritize self-care through the chaos. Retain perspective.

Join Support Groups – Nothing comforts like solidarity. Both in-person and online communities for women navigating perimenopause and menopause provide the safety net of shared experience. You don't walk alone.

Reframe Perspective – When the unforeseen changes and losses feel crushing, remind yourself this transition makes space for reinvention, rest, and wisdom. New beginnings emerge.

With compassion for the process, self-nurturing, and social support, you build reserves of resilience to weather periods of uncertainty ahead. Together you'll find pearls nestled within every oyster of struggle.

Intimacy Considerations

The physical and psychological effects accompanying perimenopause often impact couples' sex lives and emotional intimacy. But proactive, creative solutions prevent connection from becoming casualty.

Vaginal dryness and discomfort frequently increase during this time thanks to waning estrogen. Without sufficient lubrication, intercourse and orgasm proves difficult or impossible. However, remedies help:

- Use silicone or water-based lubricants generously during lovemaking. Reapply as needed.

- Try longer foreplay focused on arousal. Oral sex and manual stimulation reduces reliance on penetration.

- Incorporate sex toys and vibrators to aid stimulation and pleasure when discomfort persists.

- Discuss options like topical estrogen or dehydroepiandrosterone (DHEA) if over-the-counter lubricants insufficiently help. But monitor for PCOS related side effects.

- See a pelvic floor therapist if penetrative pain continues despite lubricants. Physical therapy eases vulvodynia and vaginismus.

- Focus intimacy on whole-body sensuality, erotic massage and creative play when intercourse feels impossible. Prioritize mutual pleasure without pressuring particular acts.

Frequent open affection and praise outside the bedroom also lifts spirits making sexual intimacy flow more smoothly. Verbalize understanding around physical discomforts. If ED accompanies waning testosterone, explore aids like oral medications, pumps or supplements under medical guidance.

When libidos ebb, don't take it personally. Hormones and health issues temporarily suppress desire. However, emotional and physical closeness remains vital. Intentionally nurture non-sexual intimacy through all the uncertainties ahead. Thriving partnerships withstand storms by anchoring to each other with care.

Processing Loss and Grief

The magnitude of change this transition represents can trigger overwhelming emotions like resentment, fear, sadness, or shame. Creating space to openly process these feelings and grieve metaphorical losses breeds resilience.

Reflect together on treasured parts of youth fading away - fertility, smooth skin, stable sleep, sharp cognition, effortless fitness. Allow processing disappointment around altered curves, faces, energy levels and sex. Release expectations for this new uncharted phase.

Then look for glimmers of gained wisdom, freedom and clarity emerging through release. What possibilities and priorities feel more authentic to pursue in this season? Let go assumptions of how this stage "should" look.

When grief arises, avoid rushing your partner to positive thinking. The aim is not to "get over it", but to fully move through it. Tears and anger sometimes accompany forward growth. Through sharing vulnerability, intimacy binds you closer conquering fear.

Some thoughtful questions to prompt reflection include:

- What feelings arise as you reflect on this transition into a new stage of womanhood and partnership?

- What hopes or expectations feel most difficult to release? What helps you voice that grief?

- How do you define your identity, purpose and gifts as you evolve? What empowers you now?

- What support, changes or rituals would help you remain resilient through the ups and downs?

- How can I be a compassionate partner through the varied emotions this milestone elicits?

Let your steadying patience and perspective lift her up when the ground feels shaky. Remind her that closing one chapter simply turns the page toward rediscovered potentials.

Guiding Teens with PCOS + ADHD Through Womanhood

If you have adolescent daughters contending with both emerging womanhood and managing PCOS plus ADHD, take special care nurturing self-esteem and setting them up for health. Help them embrace their whole selves.

Given sensitivities to estrogen starting puberty, recognize mood swings or depression may intensify at this vulnerable time. Work with their psychiatrist if needed to adjust medications and therapy support. Reinforce their inherent worth often.

Since PCOS increases during adolescence, advocate for thorough diagnostic testing if irregular periods, excess hair growth, or acne appear. Early detection allows better control. But remind your daughter these traits don't define her. Celebrate her unique gifts.

Discuss healthy nutrition, activity, and sleep habits proactively, not punitively. Puberty weight changes paired with ADHD challenges require non-judgmental collaboration. Lead by your own example.

When signs of ADHD like disorganization and poor time management increase stress, show empathy. Guide creation of systems like wall calendars, alarms and checklists honoring her neurology. Share your own tips for managing executive functioning needs.

Temper social media messages tying self-worth to appearance. has... Help your daughter define beauty on her own terms beyond airbrushed influencer images. Boost diverse role models confidently rocking natural hair, curves, makeup-free skin and disability pride.

Equip your teen with resources like evidence-based websites, support groups, and mentors where she can find belonging and gain wisdom from those further along. She needs solidarity, not isolation.

Changes will come in overwhelming waves, so anchor her back to self-compassion and your unconditional love. Keep communicating and embracing her multidimensional self as she blossoms.

Relishing Restored Freedom and Fresh Perspective

While major life transitions bring growing pains, embracing midlife's liberated possibilities uplifts spirit. Let go assumptions of how this stage "should" look. Instead reinvent daily joys unique to the freedom and wisdom of your evolving chapter.

With shared humor and resilience, view unpleasant symptoms as passing inconveniences rather than identity crises. Hot flashes too will fade. Discomfort prompts creativity discovering what works for your distinctive bodies now.

When health demands seem to monopolize life, take comfort knowing this too shall pass. Menopause ushers in reclaimed time and energy as parenting duties lessen and careers plateau. Pace yourself through the intensity.

After reproductive years conclude, a sense of restoration, lightness and newfound direction often emerges. Define fulfillment by your distinctive standards, not society's narrow symbols. What genuinely feeds your spirit today?

What priorities or neglected parts of self now hold more urgency worth nourishing? How will you infuse daily purpose? Allow this transition to redirect your compass toward passions.

What growth, talents and creations will you birth amidst the empty nest? How will you nurture intimacy and community? Let this milestone reawaken your playful inner child.

Savor the bittersweet beauty of change. Each decade reveals expanded potentials. Though paths meander unexpectedly at times, trust it ultimately guides you home to your most authentic selves.

Navigating PCOS, ADHD, and menopause in parallel provides unique challenges, yet simultaneously cultivates resiliency and wisdom. Consistent self-care, community support, perspective, and teamwork smooth the transition.

This natural progression invites you to release limiting assumptions and defining strength through flexibility. By honoring the grieving process, you make space for the growth continuing change brings.

Your power always remains choice - at every age and stage - to view life through a lens of gratitude, possibility, and meaning. Use challenges as catalysts to unearth latent potentials, priorities and courage.

Have faith that the sun keeps rising through night skies. Dance with your ever-evolving rhythms. Though aging brings poignant losses, upstairs new rooms you've yet to discover also await. Keep climbing. The view widens.

Cultivating Mental Health and Coping Skills

Between racing thoughts, emotional sensitivity, executive functioning challenges, and the stigma surrounding neurodiversity, those contending with ADHD and PCOS often confront steep mental health hurdles. Intentionally nurturing your mental wellbeing proves essential.

Let's explore strategies including helpful thought patterns, stress management skills, therapeutic outlets, social support, and professional help for constructing mental resilience on tough days. You deserve to feel empowered in your mind and spirit while navigating these diagnoses.

Managing Inner Critic Conversations

"I should be able to focus better." "I'm so lazy and undisciplined." The inner critic's constant judgments erode confidence and self-care motivation when living with ADHD. Begin noticing and redirecting its fixed negative narrative.

Tune Into Self-Talk – Recognize instances when your inner voice shames your symptoms as moral failures. These comments often start with "I should..." or focus on exaggerating your flaws.

Get Curious – When you catch critical self-talk arising, gently investigate where these patterns originated. Did someone important once label you this way? Does society narrowly define normalcy? Unpack the roots without judgment.

Reframe from Deficit to Difference – Challenge internal comments like "Something is wrong with my brain" by reframing ADHD as neurodiversity - simply a different thinking style with unique strengths. Deficits become differences.

Speak to Yourself as a Friend – If harsh criticisms arose in your mind, pause and reflect how you would respond to a loved one struggling. Treat yourself with that same compassion and understanding.

Replace "Shoulds" – Whenever expectations like "I should be able to muscle through this fatigue" arise, restate affirmations about your inherent worth not depending on tasks completed. Release rigid demands of yourself.

Focus on Progress – Counteract perfectionism and failure fixation by proactively listing daily accomplishments, acts of self-care, or instances you implemented a helpful strategy. Celebrate all growth.

Set Loving Goals – Establish supportive goals framed positively around adding in behaviors that make you feel nourished and empowered rather than depriving objectives fueled by self-criticism. Love attracts love.

Respond to the inner critic with the same gentle guidance you would provide a friend struggling. Your mental health flows from self-acceptance, not self-blame.

Working Through Anxiety, Worry and What-Ifs

The uncertainty and overwhelm accompanying chronic health conditions understandably breed anxiety for the future. However, excessive worry wastes precious present moments. Ground against fretting "what ifs" by:

Questioning Worries – Is this a concern about something concretely happening or just an unlikely hypothetical scenario? Get perspective on realistic probabilities and prevent spinning unrealistic "what if" tales.

Naming Current Reality – Bring yourself back into the present by slowly noticing your direct surroundings - sights, textures, sounds, smells. Engage your senses to exit rumination.

Finding Gratitude – Make a running list of all current life blessings and joys that still exist right now, from basic comforts and abilities to loved ones. Abundance remains now.

Releasing Control – Ask yourself how much power you truly have over the unknown future outcomes provoking anxiety. Redirect energy toward embracing the gifts of today.

Writing It Down – Free your mind by emptying worries onto paper then setting them aside knowing they're captured. Externalizing thoughts reduces their grip.

Breathing Through – Pause everything and spend 5 minutes taking deep diaphragmatic breaths. Anxiety lifts as you slow down and return to your body.

Talking It Out – Voice your specific worry aloud to a trusted confidant. Their reassurance and grounded perspective defuse perceived "emergency."

Making Contingency Plans – For legitimate concerns, brainstorm reasonable preparations you could make. Action reduces helplessness. Discuss options with your partner.

While imagined futures can feel threatening, emotional relief remains available here and now. When anxiety strikes, redirect attention to the safety surrounding you in the present moment.

Nurturing Peace Through Mindfulness Practices

Daily mindfulness habits provide tools regulating difficult thoughts, emotions, and sensations when they do arise. Some basics to build skills:

Breathwork – Spend 5-10 minutes twice daily focusing fully on the sensations of breathing. Let this anchor in the now calm racing minds.

Body Scans – Slowly scan attention from the top of your head down through toes, observing any areas of physical tension to release.

Walking Meditation – Take mindful slow walks letting senses fully engage - sights, sounds, smells, contact with the ground. Let nature soothe.

Mantras – Repeat centering phrases like "I am safe", "This too shall pass", "I breathe in calm" etc. to self-soothe and refocus when stressed.

Visualization – Picture serene images like floating on clouds or resting by water. Make visualizations richly sensory by incorporating sounds, smells and sensations.

Yoga – Gentle flowing sequences with focused breathing provides active mindfulness. But also try restorative poses easing tension.

Loving Kindness – Send blessings and well wishes first to yourself, then loved ones, difficult people, and the whole world. Feel empathy spread.

Start small practicing just 5-10 minutes daily. Gradually mindfulness shifts brain pathways reducing reactivity. Return to your center amidst the whirlwind.

Cultivating Emotional Wellbeing through Therapy

Chronic health conditions often profoundly impact emotional wellbeing. Seeking counseling proactively fortifies mental health before crises strike. Ongoing therapy provides:

Coping Skills – Therapists offer tools to healthily manage stress, anxiety, sadness, anger and emotional reactivity. You gain long-term life skills for self-regulation.

Insight on Patterns – Counselors help reveal unhelpful habitual thought loops and core beliefs you repeat unconsciously. Awareness brings choice.

Emotional Release – Sessions allow a safe space to vent frustrations, grief, resentment about diagnoses. Voicing feelings prevents repression into depression.

Supportive Presence – Knowing you have a regular non-judging outlet with a therapist provides comfort during life's up and down spells. Their stability anchors amid chaos.

Perspective – When caught in emotion or worry, a counselor's grounded guidance realigns with wisdom, keeping difficulties in balanced perspective. They remind you of full context.

Growth – Therapists nurture self-esteem, help set health-promoting goals and walk with you through progress and setbacks alike. They believing in your innate strengths.

Treatment Synergy – Counseling helps maximize lifestyle measures and medical treatments for PCOS and ADHD working in parallel. Holistic care catalyzes growth.

Make therapy sessions both a means of receiving support during current struggles and an investment in long-term mental health resilience. The stronger your emotional core, the more empowered you feel navigating all of life's twists and turns.

Self-Care Inspiring Mental Wellness

Consistent nurturing self-care habits provide the foundation uplifting mental health. However, don't let busyness become a barrier. Take actions speaking that you matter.

Move Daily - Any joyful movement - walking, dancing, yoga, weights, etc. – releases feel-good neurotransmitters naturally. Just get moving. Play a song that moves you and start moving.

Eat Intuitively – Enjoy balanced nourishing meals and snacks as preventive medicine. Don't restrict or emotionally eat. Notice how food choices impact your mind.

Hydrate Well – Dehydration exacerbates cognitive dysfunction and mood issues. Sip fluids consistently, especially water and herbal tea. Carry a bottle as a visual cue.

Sleep Deeply - Prioritize 7-9 hours nightly, wind down effectively, and keep bedrooms cool and comfy for restorative rest. Protect sleep consistency.

Pursue Passions – Make time for hobbies that take you into a state of immersive flow. Whether music, gardening, puzzles or photography, tap into joy.

Find Your People – Surround yourself with supportive communities sharing similar struggles online and locally who "get it." Feeling understood uplifts spirits.

Set Boundaries – Limit time with draining people and obligations. Toxic energy sabotages mental health. Protect your inner light. You teach people how to treat you.

Detox Digital – Unplug blocks of time daily for activities offline nourishing the spirit like reading, creating, walking, chatting with loved ones. Regulate exposure.

Counsel Carefully – Seek a therapist skilled in ADHD, chronic health emotional needs, and holistic support beyond just medication. Ensure an empowering fit.

Through ongoing self-care, you proactively build mental reserves protecting against depletion long-term. Nurture your whole being.

Utilizing Inspiring Outlets and Tools

Certain therapeutic outlets and modalities also nurture emotional wellbeing in uplifting ways. Explore adding in:

Gratitude Journaling – Keep an actual or digital journal where you record a few things daily you feel grateful for. Cultivate awareness of goodness surrounding you.

Stream of Consciousness Writing – Empty racing thoughts, worries or creative ideas onto paper through free associative journaling. Let the mind wander without censor to calm inner noise.

Art and Music Therapy – Express emotions through painting, drawing, clay sculpting, dance/movement, learning instruments, listening to or making playlists. Creativity heals.

Nature Immersion – Absorb the soothing benefits of fresh air, greenery, sunlight, and animals by spending time walking, hiking, gardening etc. Nature restores peace.

Pet Therapy – If you don't have your own, volunteer to walk shelter dogs and play with cats. Non-judgmental furry affection relieves stress.

Talking Circles – Join a support group filling emotional needs missing in other relationships. Listen and share mutual experiences without judgement.

Mindfulness Apps – Try quality-vetted apps like Calm, Headspace, InsightTimer. They offer short accessible meditations and sleep stories managing anxiety.

Cognitive Exercises – Do puzzles, play strategy or memory strengthening games, learn new skills to build confidence while enhancing brain health.

Integrate outlets that uniquely speak to your spirit and soothe overwhelm. Explore those which feel playful and inspiring versus mandated. Follow intuition to your own medicine.

Knowing When to Seek Medication

For some with severe chronic anxiety, depression, OCD, bipolar disorder etc, psychiatric medications provide critical aid regulating brain chemistry imbalances along with counseling and lifestyle strategies. Do not hesitate seeking medication when:

- You struggle functioning from profound sadness, irrational worry, panic attacks, compulsions or mood swings

- Symptoms persist daily over 2+ weeks despite self-care and therapy

- Thoughts of self-harm, suicide, or harming others arise

- You experience disordered eating, substance abuse or severe social withdrawal

- Psychosis emerges - detachment from reality, paranoia, hallucinations

- Previously manageable symptoms become highly disruptive to relationships, work, health

Speak openly with your prescriber about all symptoms impairing quality of life. With patience fine-tuning formulations and dosage, medications allow you to thriving fully. They treat mental health conditions just like any other illness.

While gauging effectiveness, track benefits and any side effects needing attention like sleep changes, appetite shifts or fatigue. Jot down mood, sleep and diet daily. Frequent follow up lets providers optimize treatment.

Medication facilitates functioning, not fundamental life change alone. It works best alongside counseling, community support and healthy routines. But never hesitate utilizing it as part of your toolbox when needed.

Relating Skillfully with Friends and Family

ADHD and chronic health struggles inevitably shape social relationships. Certain communication approaches help foster understanding from friends and family when tensions arise.

Share Resources – Provide loved ones informative articles, books, documentaries and social media accounts illuminating your diagnoses. Increased knowledgeoften builds empathy. Let them into your world.

Explain Your Experiences – Don't just list symptoms and treatment facts. Help loved ones grasp how ADHD and health conditions impact you emotionally – the losses, fatigue, wins, confusion and courage navigating it all. Share you.

Ask How They Feel – Check in about loved ones' honest thoughts and concerns regarding your diagnoses. Addressing unspoken worries prevents rifts from growing silently. Give space for their processing too.

Teach Through Modeling – Demonstrate what supportive responses sound like when you hit obstacles. Your calm handling of setbacks models resilience for family and friends.

Set Kind Boundaries – If loved ones say hurtful or dismissive things out of ignorance, gently but firmly explain the damage caused while offering education. Just beware lecturing.

Focus on Shared Humanity – Relate to others on universal commonalities - hope, purpose, meaning, relationships. Illness represents just one dimension of the whole you and others.

Give it Time – Remember growth and learning happen gradually. Allow loved ones space getting familiar with changes in you and your dynamic. Meet defensiveness with patience.

Let Go with Love – If certain relationships remain toxic despite communication efforts, know when to peacefully release contacts continuously wounding your spirit. Cherish those who nurture you.

Through compassion, education and insight into each other's inner worlds, build deeper mutual understanding with those you hold dear. Shared empathy connects.

Redirecting from Guilt into Empowerment

The enormity of navigating dual diagnoses risks burdening you with disempowering guilt. Counter these thoughts by getting radically honest about the aspects actually within your control:

Allow room for grief - Recognize mentally bargaining or blaming yourself cannot erase loss or hardship. Giving sorrow its full space enables eventual acceptance.

Release regretting the past - Judging past actions as foolish prevents serving your current needs. Reflect for insights but don't letcould-haves overshadow the possibilities ahead.

Face fears - Worrying obsessively cannot control the future. Shift energy into contingency planning and creating stability day by day within your reach . You have more power than you realize.

Accept existing limits - Beating yourself up over perceived inadequacies or failures exhausts spirit. We all navigate challenges differently. Release rigid standards.

Get curious about stories - Question overly simplistic inner narratives of yourself as victim or saboteur. See the nuance. External and genetic factors always influence health.

Take radically responsibility - While you can't control everything, seize initiative over daily actions, thoughts and choices promoting your wellbeing. Don't become passive.

Know your worth - Regret implies you are unworthy as you are. But no error revokes your beauty and inherent value. You cannot earn worthiness - it exists in your essence.

Find meaning - Seek inspiring communities and fulfilling outlets like volunteering, creating, exploring where your diagnoses intersects with purpose. Healing arises by sharing gifts.

Stay grounded in realistic humility. By boldly separating guilt from growth, you walk forward with agency. Write a new chapter.

A Journey of Love, Understanding, and Growth

When your partner received a diagnosis like ADHD or PCOS, it likely opened up a well of questions and worries about this unexpected fork in your planned road. Confronting chronic health conditions and neurodiversity can certainly reroute hopes for how life and partnership might unfold.

Yet in retrospect, those points of divergence ultimately directed you down routes of insight you'd never have encountered otherwise. What first felt like an obstacle blinded you to the steep learning and rapid personal growth awaiting discovery once you adjusted lens and expectations.

While each couple's story proves unique, over time certain themes emerge as beacons guiding couples forward with renewed faith when the terrain grows rough:

- Patience – Progress flows steadily through small daily actions compounded over years, not instant overnight transformation. Trust in incremental steps when change feels perpetual.

- Perspective – Challenges appear insurmountable when focused on up close. Zoom out to recognize how far you've already come and the hopeful strides made. Where there is life, there are possibilities.

- Flexibility – Rigid assumptions about what "should be" at certain ages or stages only breed disappointment. Release timelines. Meet each season and limitation with openness to redefine happiness.

- Creativity – When familiar well-worn paths no longer serve, invent new passages and solutions tailored to your unique needs and values right now. Limitation inspires innovation.

● Connection – No matter how alone or overwhelmed you may feel, thousands journey this same terrain. Seek out communities and resources bridging understanding. You never walk solo.

● Rest – Demanding conditions require even more diligent self-care to prevent depletion. Give yourself permission to retreat and recharge through it all. Progress isn't linear.

● Gratitude – In the midst of hardship and uncertainty, purposefully notice daily gifts - having a roof overhead, hot coffee, music, laughter, sunshine. Count blessings over burdens.

● Empathy – Rather than judging your partner's differences, open your heart to truly understanding how ADHD and PCOS shape thoughts, emotions and behaviors from the inside out. Insight breeds compassion.

● Purpose – Whether through work, parenting, art, or volunteering in your community, continually reconnect to activities feeling meaningful and uplifting. Small daily purpose compounds to hope.

● Presence - Anxiety about the future threatens our ability to fully engage the only certain moment - this one. Breathe deeply and bring full focus to the blessings immediately surrounding you.

Your power always remains in your openness to learn, adapt, and lean into community and perspective expanding possibilities when diagnoses feel limiting at first. But in fact, these roads opened up vistas your old path never could have.

While ongoing management means this healing journey lasts a lifetime, fear and uncertainty learned to make space for empathy, intimacy and renewed purpose when you adjusted expectations. Rather than cursing storms, you learned to dance in the rain.

Of course there are still slippery slopes and backward slides when symptoms flare or mutually supportive communication goes awry. Not every day includes profound growth or giddy joy. This is the reality of any lifelong partnership.

Yet on the days when diagnoses feel like ruthless taskmasters, remind yourselves how many mountains you've already crested as a team. Hold on to warm memories of victories large and small - finishing a 5k hand-in-hand, laughing through Attempt 50 at perfecting your chocolate soufflé recipe, tearful baby cuddles at 3am.

These are the sacred moments that thread together to tell a story wilder and more wonderful than either of you could have dreamed.

So take a deep breath whenever the present feels too painful or frightening. This too shall evolve. Your history stands testament. Come back to the last thing that made you belly laugh or proudly think "I chose the right partner." Return to the light you've birthed through every previous dark night. It will come again. It always does.

You Have All You Need For The Path Ahead

May you remember that you already hold every resource within to navigate each rise and dip with wisdom, courage and joy. At times you'll need patience most of all - with your partner, yourself, friends who don't fully understand your reality. Many will only be able to grasp half the picture. That's ok. You see the full beauty.

On days your partner especially wrestles with shame, anxiety or discouragement, take their face lovingly in your hands and remind them they are worthy and empowered. They are wildly more than random neurons misfiring or hormones gone haywire. Their essence always remains whole. Help them unlock the cage of limiting stories.

Some periods, your most heroic act involves simply putting one foot in front of the other when all feels impossibly overwhelming. Forgive small lapses. Progress comes in waves, including healthy rest and retreat when depleted. Nourish yourself first so you can fully nourish each other.

Through it all, maintain faith in your ultimate resiliency as individuals and as a team. Hardship pulls back the bow launching your personal potential ever forward. Heartache serves to make room for unexpected fulfillment. Suffering builds spiritual stamina. What you have endured already, you can endure again with grace.

You each prove far more powerful and courageous than any diagnosis could ever define you. Let strength and wisdom unfold one merciful day at a time. Keep watering the seeds of knowledge, community, resilience and love - they promise fruits in due season you can't yet imagine. You've made it this far. Now breathe, and carry on together.

The Light Always Returns

Darkness always births the light again. Seasons cycle progressing humanity's journey generation after generation. The sun never ceases rising.

So take heart during phases that feel bleak and interminable. They will pass. Dawn breaks again. Vibrant chapters lie ahead.

Until then, kindle small steady flames - love notes left on pillows, hands held during doctor visits, friends who understand, restorative nature walks, and therapeutic laughter. Keep stoking your inner hearth.

The sun returns gradually, not instantly. But it always circles back. Trust in eventual joy; it waits to reveal your wisdom gained through plodding uphill. New perspective ripens your readiness to receive blessings you'd have formerly overlooked in rush.

Can you look back now and see how this unexpected path held treasures you'd have missed if life came easily? Did your creativity, compassion, priorities, and passions deepen? That's often growth's sweet paradox - digging through mud uncovers hidden gold.

What friends, communities, and inner strengths emerged you'd never have recognized without this catalyst of change? Which relationships and old mindsets naturally released to make space for more vibrant new shoots?

There is light if you look for it. But you must trust its arrival as much in times of monsoon downpour as in sunny seasons. It appears differently across moments, requiring an adjusted gaze - light as love notes left on pillows, patience exchanges, friends who understand, restorative nature walks, and therapeutic laughter. But the light always remains if you know where to look for its arrival.

It gradually returns through simple consistent actions - waking to journal gratitudes, preparing nutritious meals amidst fatigue, choosing to belly laugh when you want to cry, reaching for your partner's hand in the waiting room, whispering hopes instead of frustrations before sleep. These become the steady subtle sources illuminating each next step among seeming uncertainties.

So stoke the inner hearth with forgiveness, faith and vulnerability. Protect its fragile but certain flame. Joy will come when you tend yourself and each other with care enough to wait out the darkness.

For now, bundle up with blankets heavy and nurturing as community support, hot tea, and rest. Let it replenish and warm you for the waiting. This too shall pass. Hold on.

References and Further Reading

ADHD and PCOS represent complex conditions warranting deep compassion, education, and support. For readers seeking to expand their knowledge and community, a wealth of helpful resources exist both in traditional media and online.

Books

- Taking Charge of Adult ADHD by Russell Ramsay and Anthony Rostain (Routledge, 2015)

- The ADHD Effect on Marriage by Melissa Orlov (Plantain Press, 2010)

- 8 Keys to Parenting Children with ADHD by Cindy Goldrich (W.W. Norton & Company, 2020)

- The PCOS Workbook by Angela Grassi and Stephanie Mattei (New Harbinger, 2019)

- Period Repair Manual by Lara Briden (HarperOne, 2017)

- PCOS for Dummies by Gaynor Bussell and Sharon Perkins (Wiley Publishing, 2020)

- The Insulin Resistance Solution by Rob Thompson and Dana Carpender(Fair Winds Press, 2016)

ONLINE

- ADDitudeMag.com – Articles, advice, and support for living with ADHD across the lifespan

● PCOS Diva - Articles and coaching on all aspects of navigating PCOS holistically

● SoulCysters.com – Forum community sharing a wide range of PCOS experiences

INSTAGRAM COMMUNITIES

Some particularly inspiring Instagram accounts uplifting those with ADHD and PCOS include:

@ADHD_Love – Fostering relationships impacted by ADHD with education and compassion

@The.Holistic.Psychologist – Science-based tools for mental health empowerment

@ThePCOSDietitian - Nutrition and lifestyle guidance specific to balancing PCOS

@PCOS.Nutritionist – Advice on managing PCOS through personalized nutrition support

The digital world allows those navigating dual diagnoses to always access compassion, feel understood, and gain practical wisdom through shared experiences. Exploring these science-backed resources equips readers to thrive while building a supportive tribe.

I'm sure there are more out there.

Find the ones that speak to you.

Don't miss out!

Visit the website below and you can sign up to receive emails whenever Bradley Hall publishes a new book. There's no charge and no obligation.

https://books2read.com/r/B-A-SCSZ-BUPOC

BOOKS 2 READ

Connecting independent readers to independent writers.

Did you love *Embracing Complexity: Understanding PCOS and ADHD in Relationships*? Then you should read *The Enneagram and Money*[1] by Bradley Hall!

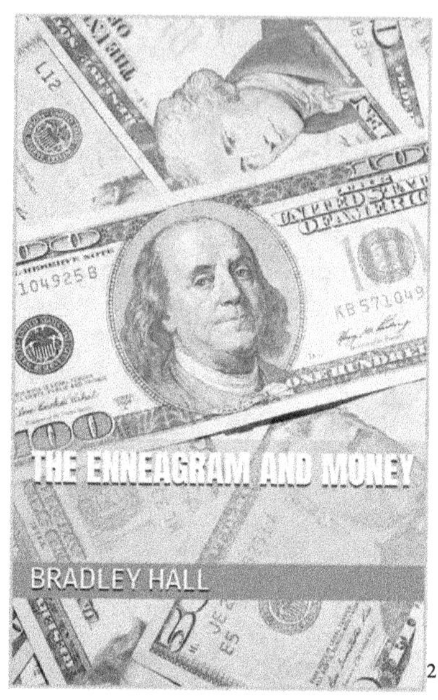

[2]

Unlock the secrets to financial empowerment with this in-depth exploration of the Enneagram and money. This groundbreaking book delves into the core motivations, fears, and unconscious patterns of each Enneagram type and how they influence financial behaviors. Discover how your personality shapes your relationship with money and gain profound insights to transform limiting financial patterns.

Through fascinating explorations of each type, from the Perfectionist to the Peacemaker, this book provides a roadmap to align your values, passions, and actions with your financial life. Overcome self-sabotaging behaviors, cultivate abundance and gratitude, and make conscious money choices that pave the way to genuine fulfillment and prosperity.

---

1. https://books2read.com/u/3GGpJr

2. https://books2read.com/u/3GGpJr

Within these pages, finance expert Bradley Hall blends their expertise in Enneagram personality types and financial dynamics to offer practical tips and exercises tailored to your unique needs. This allows you to leverage your natural strengths, overcome weaknesses, and establish financial balance and well-being.

Whether you're an Enneagram enthusiast or simply seeking financial wisdom, this book provides invaluable tools to master your money mindset. By embracing your core motivations and integrating your personality with your financial goals, you can embark on a transformative journey to financial authenticity and abundance.

Also by Bradley Hall

The Enneagram and Money
Why Won't My Children Talk to Me? A Book For Conservatives
Embracing Complexity: Understanding PCOS and ADHD in Relationships

About the Author

Bradley Hall lives in Raleigh, North Carolina with his wife, Amanda, and their dog Yelena.

Bradley is an enrolled agent and tax expert who took on the task of writing this book to help himself with his wife's dual diagnosis of PCOS and ADHD, both still mostly misunderstood medical disorders.

He hopes that this book will help those who either battles these dual disorders and those who live with them.

www.ingramcontent.com/pod-product-compliance
Lightning Source LLC
Chambersburg PA
CBHW050803260726

48660CB00004B/1226